THE TROPICAL MEDICINE HANDBOOK QUESTIONS & ANSWERS

Dr. Benjamin Alli is a Sakellarides Professor of Medicine & Surgery and the Chancellor of theRoyal College of Physicians and Surgeons of the United States of America.

Published By: **Elite Exclusivity**
Edited By: **Mugheer Ahmad**

Introduction by: Dr. Christopher Smithmyer

Elite exclusivity

Dysart Detroit Dallas

Send all Inquiries to: EliteExclusivityPR@gmail.com,
and Info@EliteExclusivity.com

First Edition

ISBN Paperback: 978-1-952651-06-9
ISBN Hardback: 978-1-952651-12-0

Printed in the United States of America

Table of Contents

Introduction

Nietzsche once said that "if you stare into the abyss the abyss will stare back into you." The meaning of this statement is that if you look into something so unfathomable as the abyss, it will change you as a person and show you what is present inside your soul. The same can be said for if you stare into the mind of a genius, this process will forever change how you see the world around you. I have had this privilege in doing the review of this work by Dr. Benjamin Alli, seeing the functions and the functionality of one of the great minds of our time has allowed me a deeper understanding into medicine, although I am not a medical doctor.

The *Tropical Medicine Handbook* is a utility belt of sorts. Dr. Alli looks at individual questions from the field and addresses them as he feels they need address. Some questions are addressed with a simple sentence, others are addressed with pages of diagnostic notes. To each question he affords the space needed, no less no more. Some of the questions are answered in technical language, some in carefully sorted prose, yet others with outlines or charts to help the reader walk through a greater understanding of the answer as can only be taught by a master at work.

Understanding where the ideas came from is not as important as understanding where the data comes from. With a lifetime of experience, Dr. Alli is both the writer and the source for some of the answers. The specific citations can be found in his voluminous works, but where he reaches beyond his own expertise, there is a set of citations at the end of each section. This allows the reader to distinguish between what is written by the sage and what is written by other experts in the field.

Mastery of a field, at least at this level, is a curious thing. We are privileged to live in a time where this information can be recorded and documented, becoming part of the international canon before it is lost to time like so much other great knowledge. The format is challenging as it changes to meet the needs of each question; however, the depth of understanding to be gained through out these pages is worth the challenge as you delve into Dr. Benjamin Alli's masterwork, *The Tropical Medicine Handbook: Questions and Answers.*

- Dr. Christopher W. Smithmyer

What is *The Tropical Medicine Handbook: Questions and Answers*?

The Tropical Medicine Handbook is a reference guide that provides information on various medical topics and conditions. While this was written with healthcare professionals such as doctors, nurses, and medical students in mind, patients and their families may find it useful as well.

It covers a broad range of topics related to medicine, including anatomy, physiology, pharmacology, diagnosis, treatment, and management of various medical conditions. There is also information on medical procedures, laboratory tests, and medical equipment. Many of these questions came up frequently throughout my medical journey.

While medications, recommendations and general practice should be cross referenced with health professionals before diagnosing and treating patients, *The Tropical Medicine Handbook* can be used as a quick reference guide to quickly access important information. They may also be used by patients and their families to better understand their medical conditions and treatment options.

Question 1 Discuss the role of genetic factors as the cause of human disease.

Genetic factors play an essential role in the cause of human diseases. Genetic factors can bebroadly classified as follows: -

Single gene defects (Mendelian) - This type of genetic disorder has a clear inheritance pattern (autosomal or sex-linked), dominant or recessive, and presents as a high risk to the relatives. Someexamples:

- Autosomal dominant: Achondroplasia, Adult polycystic disease, Huntington's chorea, Neurofibromatosis.
- Autosomal recessive: Cystic fibrosis, Friedreich's ataxia, Hemochromatosis, Sickle cellanemia.
- Sex-linked recessive: Duchenne muscular dystrophy, Fragile X syndrome, Sex-linked dominant: Vitamin D-resistant rickets

Chromosomal genetic disorders - This type of genetic disorder could result from the loss, gain or abnormal rearrangement of one or more of the 46 chromosomes in the diploid cell. It has no clear inheritance pattern and presents as a low risk to the relatives. Some examples:

1. Autosomal disorders: Trisomy 21 (Down's syndrome), Trisomy 13 (Patau's syndrome Trisomy 18 (Edwards' syndrome)
2. Sex chromosome disorders: Fragile X syndrome (46, XX), Turner's syndrome (45, XO),

Klinefelter's syndrome (47, XXY).

c) Multifactorial genetic disorders - This type of genetic disorder is due to the interaction between genes and environmental factors and presents as a low risk to the relatives. Some examples: Hypertension, schizophrenia, neural tube defects, pyloric stenosis, ankylosing spondylitis, cleft palate, alcoholism, diabetes mellitus, epilepsy, manic-depressive psychosis, coronary heart disease, and thyroid disease.

d) Mitochondrial genetic disorders - This type of genetic disorder is transmitted through the maternal line due to mutations in the mitochondrial genome. Some examples: Myoclonic epilepsy with ragged red fibers (MERRF), mitochondrial encephalopathy, lactic acidosis, stroke-like episodes (MELAS), and Lieber's optic atrophy.

e) Genetic factors in oncogenesis or somatic mutations that lead to malignant transformation are acquired during the person's lifetime. The molecular basis underlyingsuch genetic abnormalities can be divided into two types: -

- Activation of growth-promoting genes (oncogene to activated oncogene). Oncogenes are genes that can cause malignant transformation when the oncogenes are activated by point mutations, translocations, or gene amplification. Some examples:

Oncogene	Humor Tumor	Mechanism of Activation
Neu/erb-B2	Breast, Ovarian, and gastric carcinoma	Amplification
Erb-B	Breast carcinoma, glioblastoma	Amplification
Ki-ras	Lung and colon carcinomas	Point mutation
myc	Lymphomas	Amplification
N-myc	Neuroblastoma	Amplification
L-myc	Small cell carcinoma	Amplification
Bcl-2	Follicular and undifferentiated lymphomas	Chromosomal translocation

(ii) Tumor Suppressor Genes: Suppressor genes act by inhibiting cell growth, and a related category of genes can act by inducing apoptosis (programmed cell death). The inactivation of tumorsuppressor genes that normally suppress cell proliferation will result in tumorigenesis. Some examples:

Chromosome	Name	Types of Tumors
3p	FHIT	Small cell carcinoma and adenocarcinoma of the lung,

		cervical carcinoma renal carcinoma, von Hippel-Lindau disease
5q	APC(FPC)	Familial polyposis coli, colorectal carcinoma
11p	WT-1	WT-1 Wilm's tumor, rhabdomyosarcoma, breast carcinoma,hepatoblastoma, transitional cell bladder carcinoma, lung carcinoma.
13q	RB-1	Retinoblastoma, osteosarcoma, ductal breast carcinoma, bladder carcinoma
13q	BRCA-2	Breast carcinoma in both males and females
17p	P53	Small cell lung carcinoma, colorectal carcinoma, breast carcinoma, osteosarcoma, squamous cell lung carcinoma
17q	BRCA-1	Breast carcinoma, ovarian carcinoma, and breast-ovariancarcinoma syndrome
17q	NF-1	Neurofibromatosis type 1 (von Recklinghausen NF)
18q	DCC	DCC Colorectal carcinoma
22q	-	Neurofibrom atosis type 2, acoustic neuroma, pheochromo cytoma

References:

1. Harrison's Principles of Internal Medicine - 13th Edition
2. Medicine International (January 1994); Volume 22:1

Question 2 How would you classify pneumonia?

Consider classifying pneumonia based on:

A. Infecting Agent:

1. Bacterial Pneumonia:

a. Pneumococcal- Streptococcus pneumoniae

b. Staphylococcal- Staphylococcus aureus

c. Streptococcal- Streptococcus pyogenes

d. Klebsiella- Klebsiella pneumoniae

e. Influenzal- Hemophilus influenzae

f. Legionella- Legionella pneumophila

g. Other bacteria- i. Coliforms- pseudomonas, proteus, Escherichia coli ii. Plague-Pasteurella pestis iii. Anthrax-Bacillus anthracis iv. Tularemia- Pasteurella tularensis v. Brucella- Brucellaspecies vi. Meningococci- Neisseria meningitidis vii. Salmonella- Salmonella typhi viii. Cysticfibrosis- Pseudomonas aeruginosa ix. Coxiella Brunetti- in abattoir X. Chlamydia psittaci- contact with birds xi, Chlamydia pneumonia - community-acquired pneumonia

h. Aspiration Pneumonia- due to

aspiration of the gastric contents or

infectedmaterial from the oropharynx

into the bronchial tree.

i. Neonatal Pneumonia- due to inhalation of

amniotic fluid in the first 48 hours andafter

48 hours to the first month of life due to

bacteria previously identified for adults.

j. Caseous Bronchopneumonia- tuberculosis.2.

Viral and Mycoplasma Pneumonia:

a. Influenza- A and B strains.
b. Measles and giant cell pneumonia.
c. Cytomegalovirus.
d. Adenovirus infection
e. Chickenpox, smallpox, and vaccinia
f. Viral infection of infancy-
Respiratory syncytial virus infection,
Coxsackie,Herpes simplex.
g. Mycoplasma pneumonia
h. Pertussis

3. Rickettsia Pneumonia

a. typhus
b. Q fever and psittacosis

4. Fungal Pneumonia:

a. Phycomycetes- Mucor mycosis and coccidioidomycosis
b. Fungi imperfect- aspergillus, blastomycosis, histoplasmosis, sporotrichosis moniliasis.

5. Chemical Pneumonia

a. Due to inhaled or ingested

chemicals, e.g., chlorine, cadmium, and

paraquat.

b. 6. Lipid Pneumonia: -

a. Due to Exogenous Inhaled fat or oily

substances, e.g., liquid paraffin or fat in food.

7. Embolic Pneumonia-

Due to blood-borne infection, that is, Pyaemia- generalized pyemia with multiple abscesses in thelung and Septic infarction- Single or multiple septic infarcts which consolidate to form pneumonic consolidation and lung abscesses.

8. Lung Abscess: -

a. Aspiration of infected material, e.g., teeth and foreign bodies.
b. Pulmonary infection.
c. Blood-borne from pyemic abscesses and septic infarcts.

B. Pneumonia in the Immunocompromised: -

Due to AIDS, lymphomas, leukemias, use of cytotoxic drugs and corticosteroids.
a. Pneumocystis carinii
b. Actinomyces israelii
c. Nocardia asteroids
d. Cytomegalovirus
e. Aspergillus fumigatus

C. Anatomical Distribution of the Consolidation:

1. Lobar Pneumonia is caused by a. Pneumococci- mainly

b. Klebsiella bacilli c. Beta-hemolyticstreptococci d. Staphylococci e. Legionella

2. Bronchopneumonia is caused by a. Staphylococci b. Streptococci c. Hemophilus influenza d.Pneumococci e. Viruses f. Tuberculosis g. Other organisms of low pathogenicity

References:

1. Harrison's Principles of Internal Medicine - 13th Edition.
2. Davidson's Principles and Practice of Medicine-17th Edition.

Question 3 Differentiate typical pneumococci lobar pneumonia from primary atypical pneumonia(viral).

Typical Pneumococci Lobar Pneumonia	Primary Atypical Pneumonia (viral)
A. Etiology: Pneumococcus (Streptococcus pneumonia)	Influenza (discussion based mainly on it) Others: Respiratory syncytial virus, measles,varicella, and cytomegalovirus.
B. Clinical setting: Community pneumonia patients are usually previously fit.	Epidemics and pandemics are usually in the fallor winter. Influenza A and B are clinically indistinguishable infections. Influenza C is usually a minor illness.
C. Clinical features Maior's complaints: - Severe pleuritic pain and dyspnea. The chest pain can be so painful that the patient tries to splint the affected side. Thus, the respirations become shallow, rapid, and grunting with dilatation of	Acute onset with dominant headache, m malaise, muscular aches, chills, fever, nasal stuffiness, substernal soreness, and nausea. There may be a non-productive cough, sore throat, and coryza. High fever for 3 to 5 days.There may be signs of conjunctivitis,

the alae nasi. Productive cough with pinkish 'rusty' sputum. The sustained high temperature of 39 to 40.5 deg C and mildly cyanotic appear acutely ill, but vomiting, nausea, malaise, and headache are notdominant. Late untreated fatal cases include severe cyanosis, dyspnea, tachycardia, and extensive pulmonary involvement. Physical findings: Restricted movement of theaffected chest wall. The trachea has deviated away from the affected side may be due to pleural effusion or empyema. Dull percussion notes due to pleural effusion. Vocal resonance is increased, and bronchial breath sound is in established consolidation with fine basal rales.	posterior pharyngeal congestion, and a flushed face.
D. Investigations: 1. Gram staining of sputum: - Gram-positive diplococci. 2. Cultures of sputum, blood, and pleural fluid, 3. Counter immunoelectrophoretic of sputum, urine, and serum for pneumococcal	1. Leukopenia in the blood picture. 2. The virus may be isolated from the throat washings by inoculating embryonated eggs or cell cultures. Complement-fixing antibodies and hemagglutination-inhibiting antibodies couldbe detected in the second week.

antigen (more sensitive than sputum and blood cultures). Chest radiography: - shows lobar consolidation.	
E. Treatment: 1. Preferred: - Penicillin G or V(oral) Alternate: - Erythromycin, Cephalosporin.	1. Bed rest, 2. Symptomatic treatment:Analgesics, cough mixture, acetaminophen for fever. 3. Antibiotics are only for the treatment of bacterial complications. 4. Amantadine or rimantadine may be used prophylactically to decrease the duration of illness of influenza. 5. Ribavirin may be used in severelyill patients with influenza A or B.
F. Prevention: 1. Polyvalent pneumococcal vaccine (containing capsular polysaccharideantigens of 23 strains of Pneumonia) wouldbe able to lessen the severity of 85-90% of pneumococcal infections in immunocompetent patients.	1. Trivalent influenza virus vaccine may provide partial immunity up to 85% for a period of a few months to one **year.**

References:

1. Harrison's Principles of Internal Medicine – 13th Edition
2. Davidson's Principles and Practice of Medicine - 17th Edition

Question 4 List the complications which may occur with pneumococci and viral pneumonia.

Complications:

Pneumococci Pneumonia	Viral Pneumonia
1. Pulmonary Complications a. Empyema b. Pleural effusion c. Lung Abscess	1. Pulmonary Complications a. Mixed viral and bacterial pneumonia by Strep.pneumoniae, H.influenzae and Staph.aureus b. Tracheitis c. Bronchitis d. Broncholitis
2. Extrapulmonary Complications a. Bacteremia b. Endocarditis c. Pericarditis d. Herpes labialis	2. Extrapulmonary Complications a. Reye's syndrome b. Myositis, rhabdomyolysis, and myoglobinuria c. Myocarditis and pericarditis d. Encephalitis, transverse myelitis, Guillain-Barre syndrome and peripheral neuropathy e. Toxic cardiomyopathy

References:

1.Harrison's Principles of Internal Medicine - 13th Edition.

2. Davidson's Principles and Practice of Medicine - 17th Edition,

Question 5 Give treatment for staphylococcal pneumonia. Why is the prognosis poor?

Treatment for Staphylococcal Pneumonia. A. For non-penicillinase-producing strains:

1. Preferred: - Penicillin G (intravenous) or V (oral) 2. Alternative: - First-generation cephalosporins: Cefazolin IV (2g every 6 hours) for 4 to 6 weeks with or without GentamicinIV (1mg/kg 8 hourly) for 3 to 5 days.

B. For penicillinase-producing strains:

1. Preferred: - A penicillinase-resistant penicillin: Nafcillin IV (1.5g every 4 hourly) or Oxacillin IV (2.0g every 4 hourly) for 4 to 6 weeks with or without Gentamicin IV (1mg/kg 8 hourly) for3 to 5 days. (Nafcillin and Oxacillin are preferred over methicillin because of the side-effect of interstitial nephritis with methicillin). 2. Alternative: - First-generation cephalosporins Cefazolin IV (2g every 6 hours) for 4 to 6 weeks with or without Gentamicin IV (1 mg/kg 8 hourly) for 3 to 5 days.

C. For Methicillin-resistant strains:

Vancomycin IV (15mg/kg every 12 hours) for 4 to 6 weeks with or without Gentamicin IV(1mg/kg 8 hourly) for 3 to 5 days.

The prognosis is poor for Staphylococcal Pneumonia because:

The mortality rate for staphylococcal pneumonia is more than 25% compared to the overall mortality rate for pneumonia which is about 5%. 1. Patients who die from pneumonia usually have notreceived the appropriate antibiotics in sufficient dosages before or during the early stages of hospital admission. Severe community-acquired pneumonia has a high mortality, especially in those over 65 years. 2. Patients with a respiratory rate of more than 30/ min, a diastolic blood pressure of less than 60 mmHg, and blood urea of more than 7 mmol/ liter indicate a poorer prognosis and the need for intensive care. Approximately 50% of these patients who need intensive care will die. 3. Patients with bacteremia secondary to staphylococcal pneumonia maydie within 12 to 24 hours with high pyrexia, tachycardia, cyanosis, and vascular collapse. The disease may disseminate slowly, with hectic pyrexia and metastatic abscess formation in the brain, lungs, myocardium, kidneys, spleen, bones, and other organs.

4. Endocarditis is another important complication of staphylococcal bacteremia, especially among drug addicts. The mitral and the aortic valves could be damaged and involve valve rings andmyocardial abscesses. The presence of infection of the aortic valve, severe congestive heart failure, and involvement of the central nervous system indicates a poor prognostic sign. The mortality rateis 20 to 30%. Staphylococcal bacteremia may involve the tricuspid valve in drug addicts and involvement with septic pulmonary emboli. The mortality rate is 2 to 10%.

Question 6 Differentiate between joint pains of sub-acute rheumatic fever and non-rheumatic 'growing pains.'

The differentiation between joint pains of sub-acute rheumatic fever and non-rheumatic'growing pains' are:

Joint pains of Sub-acute Rheumatic Fever:

There is migratory polyarthritis in 85% of the cases. The large joints of the extremities are the most commonly affected. There may be arthritic involvement in the hands and feet. The spine, sternoclavicular and temporomandibular joints are uncommonly involved. The arthritis of large joints is often multiple and symmetrical with the 'migratory' arthritic pattern. That is, as the pain and swelling subside in one joint, other joints tend to become involved. In the other 15% of the cases, severe joints may show inflammation simultaneously. The synovium is thickened, red, and granular and later resolves to normal. The lesions are transient and very rarely give rise to residual disability. Microscopically, Aschoff nodes, mucoid or fibrinoid degeneration are seen inthe connective tissues, and similar changes are found in the joint capsules, affected tendons, fascia, and muscle sheaths, and accompanied by a lymphocytic infiltrate.

Joint pains of Non-rheumatic 'growing pains':

The commonest association with non-rheumatic 'growing pains' is osteoarthritis or osteoarthrosis. Osteoarthrosis is an extremely common degenerative process of articular cartilage. It may occur in the joints of the young age group with any form of previous mechanical derangement, for example, trauma, congenital dislocation of the hip, or osteochondritis.Osteoarthrosis occurs spontaneously in older age groups and is thus very common above the age of 60 years. The large weight-bearing joints are usually involved, for example, the hip and knee joints with asymmetrical joint involvement and no 'migratory' arthritic pattern. Pain is common and can be severe due to the synovial reaction associated with phagocytosed fragments of the degenerated cartilage. These lesions commonly give rise to a recurrent and permanent stiff and painful joint. The loss of joint space is due to thinning of the cartilage, which shows a loss of luster and a velvety appearance. Later, the cartilage will disappear in these areas to produce ulceration and expose the underlying subchondral bone. The bone becomes thickened as a buttressing effect and extends beyond the articular margins to form bony outgrowths (osteophytes). Sometimes, the subchondral bone is not thickened in some areas, thus allowing entry of synovial fluid into the underlying bone to produce a cystic appearance on the radiograph. The end result is an articular surface denuded of cartilage and formed by a highly polished surface of the berated bone with marginal osteophytes, which may break off to form loose bodies in the joint. Microscopically, the cartilage degenerates and with losses of mucopolysaccharide ground substance. The degenerate cartilage splits along the lines of the fibers to produce fronds of degenerate cartilage (fibrillation). This cartilage falls off, and the subchondral bone becomes thickened and compact. The osteophytes at the joint margins are formed by reactive new bone. The synovial membrane may show fibrous thickening and contain small degenerate cartilage foci. At a later stage, no cartilage remains, and articulation occurs between the two faces of burned, thickened subchondral bone.

References:

1. Harrison's Principles of Internal Medicine - 13th Edition.
2. Davidson's Principles and Practice of Medicine - 17th Edition.

Question 7 Discuss the relapses following an attack of Scarlet Fever.

The relapses following an attack of scarlet fever are

uncommon due to the wide use of antibioticsfor symptomatic streptococcal infections.

The relapses can be a result of the following:

1. Local factors: - Abscess in the peritonsillar or parapharyngeal space.

2. Spread of infection from the pharyngeal wall to the deeper tissues either by

A. Direct spread

B. Hematogenous or lymphatic spread

This may result in cervical lymphadenitis, peri tonsillitis or retropharyngeal abscess, sinusitis,otitis media, meningitis, bacteremia, pneumonia, rheumatic fever, and glomerulonephritis.

<u>References:</u>

1. Harrison's Principles of Internal Medicine - 13th Edition.
2. Davidson's Principles and Practice of Medicine - 17th Edition.

Question 8 The treatment for a case of sub-acute bacterial endocarditis in which the offending organism is not known.

Treatment for a case of sub-acute bacterial endocarditis in which the offending organism is notknown is: -

Nafcillin or Oxacillin, 1.5 grams every 4 hours. Penicillin, 4 million units every 4 hours orAmpicillin, 1.4 grams every 4 hours, and Gentamicin, 1 milligram/kg every 12 hours.

If the patient is allergic to penicillin, then

Vancomycin, 1 gram every 12 hours, can be

used.

References:

1. Harrison's Principles of Internal Medicine - 13th Edition,

2. Davidson's Principles and Practices of Medicine - 17th Edition.

Question 9 Differentiate between meningococci and pneumococci meningitis.

Meningococci meningitis	Pneumococci meningitis
1. Infecting Organism: Neisseria meningitidisof groups A, B, C, Y, W-135, and others.	Streptococcus Pneumoniae
2. Transmission: Droplets	May be via head trauma, cerebrospinal fluidleaks, and sinusitis.
3. Diagnostic Importances: a. Confusion, delirium, convulsions, pyrexia, headache, and vomiting Petechial rash of the skin and mucous membrane. b. Neck and back stiffness, positive Kernig and Brudzinski sign. c. Gram-negative intracellular diplococci. e.Culture of cerebrospinal fluid, blood, and petechiae aspiration.	a. Confusion, delirium, fever, andheadache. b. Meningismus c. Gram-positive diplococci of cerebrospinal d. Fluid on Gram stain.
4. Clinical Features: a. Symptoms: - High fever, chills, headache, nausea, vomiting. Severe pain in the back, headache,	a. Symptoms: - Rapid onset of fever, headache, confusion, and delirium. Clinical features of

confusion, and delirium. Abdomen and extremities. Confusion, Clinical features of pneumonia may be delirium, convulsion, and coma in the present severe cases. b. Signs: - Neck and back stiffness, positive Kernig and Brudzinski signs. Petechiae rash from pinhead-sized to ecchymoses. Gangreneand slough in severe cases.	pneumonia may be present. No typical rash is seen. Focal neurologic deficits and cranial nerve palsies are seen.
5. Investigations a. Lumbar puncture shows a purulent a. cerebrospinal fluid (CSF), increased pressure and protein, and decreased glucose.More than 1000 cells/100ml and polymorphonuclear cell predominates and contains Gram-negative intracellular diplococci. The organisms can be demonstrated by smear or culture of the oropharynx, blood, aspirated petechiae, and CSF. b. Low fibrinogen and platelet count. Increased prothrombin time, partial thromboplastin time, and fibrin dimers. c. Latex agglutination can demonstrate capsular	a. Lumbar puncture shows an increased pressure and protein and decreased glucose. More than 100 cells/100 ml and 60% polymorphonuclear predominates and contains Gram-positive cocci. The organisms can be demonstrated by smear or culture of blood and CSF. b. Latex agglutination and counter immunoelectrophoretic can detect pneumococcal antigens in CSF

polysaccharides in CSF and urine.	
6. Complications: a. Disseminated intracellular coagulation. b. Arthritis c. Cranial nerve damage: - especially the eighth cranial nerve with resulting deafness. d. Hydrocephalus	
7. Treatment: a. Penicillin G, 24 million units/24 hours in divided doses every 4 hours. If the patient is allergic to penicillin, use Ceftriaxone, 4 grams daily. If the patient is allergicto penicillin and cephalosporin, then use Chloramphenicol, 1 gram every 6 hours. Treatment is given until the patient is afebrilefor 5 days.	a. Penicillin G, 24 million units/24 hours in divided doses every 4 hours. If the patient is allergic to penicillin, then use Ceftriaxone, 4 grams daily, or Chloramphenicol, 1.5 grams every 6 hours. If the patient has penicillin-resistant pneumococci and is resistant to third generation cephalosporins, use Vancomycin plus rifampin, 10 mg/kg every12 hours. Treatment is given for 14 days.
8. Prevention: a. Polysaccharide vaccines for meningococcal group A, C, Y and W-135. b.Prophylactic Rifampicin, 600 mg twice a	

dayfor 2 days for household contacts.	

References

1. Harrison's Principles of Internal Medicine - 13th Edition.
2. Davidson's Principles and Practices of Medicine - 17th Edition.

Question 10 Discuss the clinical picture and management of Waterhouse-Friderichsen syndromein a case of meningococcemia.

Waterhouse-Friderichsen Syndrome

Waterhouse-Friderichsen syndrome is due to overwhelming meningococcal sepsis or fulminant meningococcemia resulting in a massive bilateral adrenal hemorrhage with acute adrenal insufficiency. It may occur in about 10 to 20% of the patients with high levels of meningococcal endotoxin in circulation. The mortality rate for the patient is almost invariably fatalbefore the era of antibiotics. Most deaths occur within 24 to 48 hours of a previously healthy person, thus making this syndrome one of the most awesome characteristics of this disease.

Clinical Picture:

It is meningococcemia associated with vasomotor collapse and shock characterized by an extremely rapid downhill clinical course, with extensive hemorrhage into the skin and petechiae, and purpuric lesions enlarging rapidly, hypotension, shock, confusion, coma, and death can occur within a few hours of the onset of the symptoms. There is generalized vasoconstriction in the early precheck stage; the patient may be alert and pale, with perioral cyanosis and cold extremities. In the early stage of shock, the cardiac output will decrease, the blood pressure will fall, the mental status will decrease, and a coma may now develop. Even with supportive and aggressive management, 40 to 60% of the patients would die from cardiac failure or respiratory failure. The patients who recover may have extensive sloughing of the skin and gangrene of the digitsresulting in loss of the digits.

Management:

A. Investigations: Close supervision of patients suspected of meningococcemia for the abruptchange of clinical vasomotor collapse and shock is vital to prevent this syndrome. Early administration of antibiotics and supportive treatment for meningococcemia, with or without demonstrating the organism in the investigation, is vital to prevent this condition from occurring.

1. Gram-staining of the aspirated petechiae or the buffy coat of blood shows the gram-negativcdiplococci.
2. Cultures of the blood, spinal fluid, urine, and aspirated petechiae demonstratemeningococci.
3. Latex agglutination assay or the counter immunoelectrophoretic to detect the capsular polysaccharide of the serogroups A, B, C, Y, and W-135 in the CSF, joint fluid, serum, and urine.
4. Electrolyte imbalance: - Hyponatremia, hyperkalemia, or hypercalcemia.
5. Hypoglycemia.
6. Blood picture: - Leukocytosis and eosinophilia.
7. Simplified cosyntropin stimulation test: - to demonstrate an acute adrenal insufficiency.

B. Treatment

1. Antibiotics: Penicillin G, 24 million units/24 hours in divided doses every 4 hours intravenously. If the patient is allergic to penicillin, give Ceftriaxone, 4 grams once a day, intravenously. If the patient is allergic to penicillin and cephalosporin, give Chloramphenicol, 1gram every 6 hours.

2. Glucocorticoid replacement therapy:

Hydrocortisone, 100-300 mg intravenous, and saline immediately. Then, immediately administer hydrocortisone phosphate or hydrocortisone sodium succinate, 100 mg intravenous, and continue intravenous infusions of 50-100 mg every 6 hours for the first day. Then give the same number of infusions every 8 hours on the second day and adjust the number of infusions depending on the clinical situation. Next, give oral hydrocortisone, 10-20 mg every 6 hours when the patient can tolerate it orally, and reduce the dosage to maintenance, 10-20 mg in the morning and 5-10 mg in the evening.

3. Supportive Treatment:

Treatment of shock with volume expansion and vasopressors (dopamine). Maintenance of fluidand electrolyte imbalance and treat hypoglycemia vigorously. Prevention of respiratory complications in comatose patients. Supportive improvement of visceral perfusion in shock, withclose blood urea nitrogen and creatinine monitoring. If disseminated intravascular coagulation occurs, treatment with heparin, whole blood, or fibrinogen is used.

C. Prophylactic measures:

1. Polysaccharide vaccines for groups A, C, Y, and W-135.
2. Rifampin, 600 mg twice a day for household contacts.

References:

1. Harrison's Principles of Internal Medicine - 13th Edition.

2. Davidson's Principles and Practices of Medicine - 17th Edition.

Question 11 What are the outstanding symptoms of Brucellosis? Outline treatment for a case of acute brucellosis resulting from the ingestion of raw cow's milk.

Symptoms of Brucellosis: -

There may be an acute onset with pyrexia, chills, and sweat. The fever may be intermittent, occurring especially at night, which may become a low-grade fever for a few weeks. There maybe a headache, loss of appetite, lethargy, arthralgia, especially abdominal or back pains, and constipation, which last for a few weeks and may be the only presenting symptoms to the medical personnel. The fever may persist for years, with periods of normal temperature betweenacute attacks. Male patients may have epididymitis in 10% of the cases.

Treatment for acute brucellosis resulting from the ingestion of raw cow's milk.

A. Symptomatic treatment for headaches, aches, pains, and fever with analgesics andantipyretic medication, respectively.

B. Antibiotics: Combination regimens of two or three

antibiotics are used to prevent high relapses of the disease, about 50% when using a single antibiotic regimen. The combinations are:

- Doxycycline or tetracycline and rifampin or streptomycin (or both).
- Trimethoprim-sulfamethoxazole and rifampin or streptomycin (or both).

The immediate treatment for acute brucellosis without localized brucellosis is Doxycycline, 100mg every 12 hours orally, or Tetracycline, 30 mg/kg per day in four divided doses, orally for 3 to6 weeks, and Streptomycin, 15 mg/kg every 12 hours intramuscular for the first 2 weeks. Patients with localized brucellosis will need a longer duration of treatment with tetracyclines. If tetracycline is contraindicated, as in pregnant women or children below the age of 8 years, because of the dangers of yellowish staining of the growing teeth, then trimethoprim-sulfamethoxazole (320/1600 mg/day in divided doses) can be used. Streptomycin may cause eighth-nerve damaged. Thus, the dosage must be decreased in patients with poor renal function, and an audio, graphic study to be done before starting the treatment. Rifampin, 900 mg/day, is used inthe combination as it may improve the results when the response is poor or when complications like meningitis or endocarditis are present.

Longer courses of treatment for a few months may be needed to treat relapses, like osteomyelitisor meningitis. Abscesses should be drained to haşten recovery. Splenectomy for patients with multiple relapses and splenomegaly may prevent further relapses. Pasteurization of cow's milk isessential to prevent brucellosis.

References:

1. Harrison's Principles of Internal Medicine - 13th Edition.

2. Davidson's Principles and Practices of Medicine - 17th Edition.

Question 12 Define Salmonellosis. What treatment would you recommend?

Definition of Salmonellosis.

Salmonellosis is due to salmonellae which are Gram-negative bacilli, not encapsulated, motile byperitrichous flagella, and expressing two or more forms of H antigens. Biochemically, three species are identified, that is, a. S. typhi b. S. Para typhi and S. Cholerasuis C. S. enteritidis.

Salmonellosis can be divided into:

a. Typhoidal Salmonellosis due to S. Typhi.
b. Nontyphoidal Salmonellosis due to any other Salmonellae other than S. Typhi,

Nontyphoidal Salmonellosis can present itself as acute diarrhea, focal abscesses, septicemia, meningitis, osteomyelitis, endocarditis, mycotic aneurysm, or asymptomatic. S.paratyphi A and S. Para typhi B (S. schottmuelleri) mimic S. typhi and can cause a milder form of typhoid fever.Most of the nontyphoidal salmonellosis is caused by S. enteritidis, S. Typhimurium, S. Heidelberg, and S. Newport. In the past five years, S. enteritidis has been the most common Salmonella isolated in the United States and Europe due to infected poultry eggs and milk. Nontyphoidal salmonellosis can be transmitted to humans from domestic animals, like pets, baby chicks orducks, and turtles, and from medical products of animal origin, like carmine dye (from insects), pancreatin, bile salts, tissue extract from thyroids, adrenals, stomachs or rattlesnakes.

<u>Salmonellosis can be presented in 6 clinical syndromes:</u>

1. Typhoid and paratyphoid fever (Enteric fever)
2. Food poisoning (Gastroenteritis)
3. Enterocolitis
4. Septicemia
5. Metastatic lesions: - Osteomyelitis/septic arthritis, liver abscess, brain abscess.
6. Asymptomatic carrier state.

Persistent and severe salmonellosis is also a major problem in patients with AIDS.

<u>Treatment for Salmonellosis can be divided into treatment for typhoidal salmonellosis and nontyphoidal salmonellosis:</u>

<u>A. Typhoidal salmonellosis.</u>

<u>a.</u> <u>Antibiotics:</u> Chloramphenicol orally, 3 to 4 g/day for adults and 50 to 75 mg/kg of body weight/day for children. The drug is given for two weeks, and the dosage can be reduced to *2 g*/day and 30mg/kg, respectively, if the patient becomes afebrile, usually after the 5th day of treatment. Chloramphenicol is associated with aplastic anemia; thus, the other orally available drugs are Amoxicillin, 4 to 6 *g*/day in 4 divided doses for adults and 100 mg/kg/day for children. Trimethoprim-sulfamethoxazole (640/3200 mg) in 2 divided doses daily for adults andTrimethoprim, 185 mg/square meter of body surface area per day for children. 4- fluoroquinolone, ciprofloxacin, or ofloxacin for those aged over 17 years.

For the patients who cannot tolerate orally, Ceftriaxone, intravenously, 3 to 4g once a dayin adults for 3 days or 80 mg/kg once a day in children for 5 days. Ceftriaxone is more effectiveand rapidly acting than Chloramphenicol intravenously. Other intravenously available antibiotics are trimethoprim-sulfamethoxazole, ampicillin, cefotaxime, aztreonam, and 4- fluoroquinolones.

Patients with multi-drug resistance of S. Typhi to oral drugs then may use Ceftriaxone or4-fluoroquinolone for ages over 17 years and Ceftriaxone for children.

In patients with surgical involvement like peritonitis, the patient should have a broad antibiotic regimen to cover the facultative and anaerobic bowel flora, using Chloramphenicol,Gentamicin, and Metronidazole.

b. Surgical intervention is also necessary for bowel bleeding and perforation, reducing the mortality rate.

c. Elimination of the chronic carrier state can be difficult as the organism can harbor in the gallbladder. Treatment includes i. Antibiotics: Ampicillin or amoxicillin, 100 mg/kg/day andprobenecid, 30 mg/*kg*/day or, alternatively, trimethoprim-sulfamethoxazole (160/800 mg) twic*e*/day and rifampin 600 mg daily for 6 weeks. Or a 4 week course of 4-fluoroquinolone.

ii. Cholecystectomy may be necessary.B. Nontyphoidal

Salmonellosis.

Antibiotics are given intravenously in symptomatic patients: Ampicillin, 6 to 12 *g*/day for adults and 100 mg/kg in divided doses for children. Chloramphenicol, 2 to 4 g/day for adults and 50mg/kg for children. Alternatively, we can use Ceftriaxone for children and 4-fluoroquinolone for patients aged over 17 years.

Asymptomatic patients with nontyphoidal salmonellosis should not receive antibiotics since theactive disease may be provoked and the carriage prolonged.

Treatment for gastroenteritis in Salmonellosis gives only supportive care and fluid and electrolytereplacement. Antibiotics should not be used here as they may increase the duration of the convalescent carriage state.

Prevention of Salmonellosis: -

1. Good sanitation, like clean water supplies and proper sewage disposal.
2. Quick and swift reporting to the CDC may help contain the disease's spread.
3. Education for the carriers in food handling and their proper way of disposal of stools.
4. Vaccination: Three doses of live oral vaccine (Ty2la) may protect for several years inthe United States. Purified Vi polysaccharide vaccine, one dose available in Europe, may protect for several years. 5. Eradication of nontyphoidal Salmonellosis is more difficult as the organisms are so widely occurring in nature.

References:

1. Harrison's Principles of Internal Medicine - 13th Edition,
2. Davidson's Principles and Practices of Medicine - 17th Edition.

Question 13 Outline the treatment of Salmonella Gastroenterocolitis

Treatment of Salmonella Gastroenterocolitis

Salmonella gastroenterocolitis is a short, acute infection usually caused by S. enteritidisserotype Typhimurium. The clinical features are generally mild, lasting for 3 to 5 days, and can present with fever, malaise, cramping abdominal pain, bloody diarrhea, and vomiting. Occasionally, a cholera-like picture may be present.

Treatment is symptomatic for uncomplicated enterocolitis. There should be enough fluid and electrolyte replacement. Fever and malaise can be treated with analgesics, but salicylates should be avoided to prevent the danger of intestinal bleeding. Young children, malnourished or immunocompromised infants, severely ill patients with sickle-cell disease, and those suspected of bacteremia should betreated for 3 to 5 days with trimethoprim-sulfamethoxazole (160/800 mg) twice a day, ampicillin 100 mg/kg intravenous or orally, or ciprofloxacin, 750 mg twice a day.

If a chronic carrier state develops, then eradicating it is important using antibiotics andpossible cholecystectomy as the organism may harbor in the gallbladder. Ampicillin or amoxicillin, 100 mg/kg per day, and probenecid, 30 mg/kg per day, or Trimethoprim-sulfamethoxazole (160/800 mg) twice a day and rifampin, 600 mg once a day for 6 weeks. Or a4-week course of 4-fluoroquinolone.

References:

1. Harrison's Principles of Internal Medicine - 13th Edition.
2. Davidson's Principles and Practices of Medicine - 17th Edition.

Question 14 Describe the clinical manifestations and treatment of salmonellosis due to S. typhi (typhoid fever).

Salmonellosis due to S. typhi (typhoid fever).Clinical

manifestations:

A. Symptoms: The onset of typhoid fever can be insidious, with chills and high fever but can be sudden and abrupt in children. In the prodromal stage, there will be increasing in headache, lethargy, cough, sore throat, and fever, increasing in a stepwise pattern. There may be abdominal pain and constipation. The fever reaches a plateau in about 7 *to* 10 days, and the patient will be much more ill, exhausted, and prostrated. There may be marked constipation or 'pea-soup' diarrhea. With abdominal distension. If there are no complications, the patient's condition should improve over a period of 7 to 10 days. There may be a chance of relapse up to 2 weeks after the defervescence.

B. Signs: Physical findings in the early stages are few. In the later stage, splenomegaly, abdominal distension and tenderness, mild bradycardia, dicrotic pulse, and meningismus may appear. The rash, a pink papule 2-3 mm in diameter, can be found on the trunk, the so-called 'rose-spots' that appear in the second week of the disease and fades away in 3 to 5 days.

Treatment of Salmonellosis due to S. typhi:

A. Antibiotics: Chloramphenicol orally, 3 to 4 *g*/day for adults and 50 to 75 mg/kg of body weight/day for children. The drug is given for two weeks, and the dosage can be reduced to 2 *g*/day and 30 mg/kg, respectively, if the patient becomes afebrile, usually after the 5th day of treatment. Chloramphenicol is associated with aplastic anemia. Thus the other orally available drugs are Amoxicillin, 4 to 6 *g*/day in 4 divided doses for adults and 100 mg/kg/day for children, Trimethoprim-sulfamethoxazole (640/3200 mg) in two divided doses daily for adults, and Trimethoprim, 185 mg/square meter of the body surface area per day for children. 4-fluoroquinolone, ciprofloxacin, or ofloxacin for those aged over *17* years.

For the patients who cannot tolerate it orally, Ceftriaxone intravenously, 3 to 4 g once a dayin adults for 3 days or 80 mg/kg once a day in children for 5 days. Ceftriaxone is more effective and rapidly acting than Chloramphenicol intravenously. Other intravenously available antibiotics are trimethoprim-sulfamethoxazole, ampicillin, cefotaxime, aztreonam, and 4-fluoroquinolones.

Patients with multi-drug resistance of S. typhi to oral drugs, may use Ceftriaxone or4-fluoroquinolone for ages over 17 years and Ceftriaxone for children.

In patients with surgical involvement like peritonitis, the patient should have a broad antibiotic regimen to cover the facultative and anaerobic bowel flora, using Chloramphenicol,Gentamicin, and Metronidazole.

B. Surgical intervention is also necessary for bowel bleeding and perforation, reducing the mortality rate.

C. Eliminating the chronic carrier state can be difficult as the organism can harbor in thegallbladder. Treatment includes:

i. Antibiotics: Ampicillin or amoxicillin, 100 mg/kg/day and probenecid, 30 mg/kg/day or, alternatively, trimethoprim-sulfamethoxazole (160/800 mg) twice/day and rifampin 600 mgdaily for 6 weeks, or 4 weeks course of 4-fluoroquinolone.

ii. Cholecystectomy may be necessary.References:

1. Harrison's Principles of Internal Medicine - 13th Edition.

2. Davidson's Principles and Practices of Medicine - 17th Edition.

Question 15 What organism is responsible for

most bacteriogenic 'food poisoning' cases?

Staphylococcus aureus is the organism responsible for most bacteriogenic 'food poisoning.'

Question 16 List the various forms of and specific treatments for tularemia

Tularemia

The various forms of Tularemia are:

1. Ulcer glandular Form: This is the commonest. The is a papule on the site of inoculation. Thepapule will ulcerate and is followed by tender, suppurative lymphadenopathy. Infected material can enter the eye and causes purulent conjunctivitis with periauricular lymphadenopathy.

2. Pneumonic Form: This form presents with cough, chest pain, and pneumonia and could be accompanied by pericarditis.

3. Septicemia Form: This form presents with acute onset of fever, headache, myalgia, and shock.

Treatment of Tularemia:

Streptomycin, 0.5 g intramuscularly every 6 to 8 hours, with Tetracycline, 0.5 g orally every 6hours, is administered until 4 to 5 days after the patient becomes afebrile. If tetracycline is contraindicated, then chloramphenicol, 0.5 g orally every 6 hours, can be used.

References:

1. Harrison's Principles of Internal Medicine - 13th Edition.

2. Davidson's Principles and Practices of Medicine - 17th Edition.

Question 16 B What conditions influence the development of clinical tuberculosis?

Conditions that influence the development of clinical tuberculosis:

1. Inadequate programs for disease control worldwide.

2. Multiple drug resistance to the treatment regimen for tuberculosis due to poor compliance incompleting the course of treatment, inadequate dosages and number of tuberculous drugs used for treatment, and inadequately supervised treatment.

3. The rapid rise of the world's population of young adults is the age group with the highestmortality from tuberculosis, followed by children and adolescents.

4. Contacts with patients with smear-positive pulmonary disease.

5. Co-infection with immunocompromised patients, like AIDS patients and patients on immunosuppressive therapy.

6. Those in close contact with high-risk patients, like health workers.

7. Underprivileged populations living together in overcrowded housing and poor sanitation.

Question 17 Give the three basic principles of therapy for pulmonary tuberculosis in order of their significance.

The three principles of therapy for pulmonary tuberculosis:

1. Antituberculosis drug therapy, Specific chemotherapy for treatment for all forms of tuberculosis, and to be given to all patients with active disease.

2. Isolation of patients is no longer an important principle except isolation of patients with activedisease from young children. An initial stay in the hospital for patients who cannot be depended on to take their medications regularly and those who present with difficult therapeutic problems.

3. Surgical problems. Pulmonary resection is rarely required, but drainage of an abscessfrom the tuberculous lymph nodes or empyema may be necessary.

References:

1. Harrison's Principles of Internal Medicine - 13th Edition.
2. Davidson's Principles and Practices of Medicine - 17th Edition.

Question 18 Outline the use of antituberculosis agents in pulmonary tuberculosis.

The commonly used antituberculosis drugs are:

1. Rifampicin, orally.

Children	10-20mg/kg
Adults < 50 kg	450 mg
Adults > 50 kg	600mg

2. Isoniazid (INH), orally.

Children	10-20mg/kg
Adults	200 to 300mg
Add pyridoxine, orally	10 mg (to prevent peripheral neuropathy)

3. Ethambutol, orally. Children and adults 25mg/kg for the first 8 weeks, then 15mg/kg

4. Pyrazinamide, orally Children and adults 20 to 35 mg/kg (max 2.5g)
5. Streptomycin, intramuscularly. Children 30 mg/kg

Adults	>45 kg	1g
	<45 kg	0.75g

Ant tuberculous Regimens:

1. 6 months regimen: First 2 months - Ethambutol or

Streptomycin, INH, Rifampicin, andPyrazinamide.

Next 4 months - INH and Rifampicin.

2. 9 months regimen: First 2 months - Ethambutol

or Pyrazinamide or Streptomycin andINH and

Rifampicin, Next 7 months - INH and Rifampicin.

3.12 months regimen: For the first 2 to 3 months, twice a week - Streptomycin and INH. For thewhole 12 months - INH and Thioacetazone (150 mg) daily.

References:

1. Harrison's Principles of Internal Medicine - 13th Edition.

2. Davidson's Principles and Practices of Medicine - 17th Edition.

Question 19 Give indications of surgical resection in pulmonary tuberculosis.

Indications of surgical resection in pulmonary tuberculous are:

Pulmonary resection is rarely done as antituberculosis

chemotherapy. When used strictly to the instructed regimens is very effective in the treatment of tuberculosis except if there is a need to drain an abscess from the tuberculous lymph nodes and to drain an empyema.

Question 20 Describe the clinical features and treatment of sarcoidosis.

Sarcoidosis.

Clinical Features: Sarcoidosis occurs more often in females, with the peak incidence in the thirdor fourth decades. Bilateral hilar lymphadenopathy is an important characteristic feature that is often asymptomatic and usually detected in routine chest radiography and may be associated with mild fever, malaise, cough, dyspnea, weight loss, peripheral lymphadenopathy, and dull chest pain in some patients.

Sarcoidosis can be divided into

1. Pulmonary manifestations: The patient may have increasing effort dyspnea as the disease progresses, and in a later stage, there may be signs and symptoms of cor pulmonale.

2. Extrapulmonary manifestations:

a. Skin sarcoidosis. Erythema nodosum and bilateral hilar lymphadenopathy are found together only in sarcoidosis. Lupus pernio, commonly affecting the nose, is a diffuse bluish plaque with small papules within the swelling. Nodules, papules, and plaques are found on the face, nose, ears, and neck. In addition, annular, macular lesions with central pigmentations, widespread cutaneous popular or nodular sarcoidosis, and subcutaneous may be found.

b. Ocular sarcoidosis... Anterior uveitis - This is a

common presentation with clouding of visionand painful red eyes. It may be found in 25% of the patients. In addition, keratoconjunctivitis sicca and lacrimal gland enlargement may occur. Uveoparotid fever is a syndrome consisting of bilateral uveitis and parotid gland enlargement with, sometimes, facial nerve palsy.

c. Metabolic manifestations. Renal calculi and nephrocalcinosis due to hypercalcemia and hypercalciuria.

d. Central nervous system manifestations. It may cause chronic meninge-encephalitis with sarcoid lesions within the brain and spinal cord, peripheral neuropathy, cranial nerve palsies (especially bilateral seventh nerve palsies), or myopathy.

e. Bone and joint manifestations. Arthralgia without erythema nodosum in 5% of the cases. Bonecysts in the digits.

f. Hepatosplenomegaly.

g. Cardiac manifestations. Ventricular dysrhythmias, conduction defects, and cardiomyopathywith congestive cardiac failure may be seen.

Treatment of Sarcoidosis

Depends on the staging based on the

chest radiography and tissue

involvement:Stage I. - Bilateral hilar

lymphadenopathy alone.

Stage II. - Bilateral hilar lymphadenopathy and parenchymal involvement.

(Parenchymal involvement is usually chested radiographical diffuse reticular infiltrates and focal infiltrates, acinar shadows, nodules, and cavitation can be seen)

Stage III - Parenchymal involvement alone.

In Stages I and II, sarcoidosis usually resolves by itself spontaneously, and treatment is seldom required except in patients with persistent erythema nodosum, fever, arthralgia, or iridocyclitismay require oral corticosteroid therapy for a short period.

In Stage III, symptomatic pulmonary sarcoidosis and sarcoidosis involving the eyes or the otherorgans would need oral corticosteroids for several years. Prednisolone is 20 to 40 mg daily for 4 weeks and a maintenance dose of 7.5 to 10 mg daily or 20 mg on alternate days for 6 to 12 months.

Topical steroids can be used for patients with ocular sarcoidosis and systemic steroids for persistent hypercalcemia. The erythema nodosum may be treated with a short course of 5 to 15 mg of prednisolone for 2 weeks. In addition, myocardial and neurological manifestations of sarcoidosisand uveoparotid fever may be treated with steroids.

References:

1. Harrison's Principles of Internal Medicine - 13th Edition,
2. Davidson's Principles and Practices of Medicine - 17th Edition.

Question 21 Define shigellosis (bacillary dysentery).

Shigellosis is an acute self-limiting intestinal infection caused by any of the four species of Gram-negative non-sporing bacilli. Shigellosis is found worldwide and is more prevalent in areas with poor hygiene and overcrowding. Transmission is by the fecal-oral route. These are four species: a. Shigella dysenteriae b. Shigella flexneri c. Shigella boydii d. Shigella sonnei Allof them are enter invasive except Shigella dysenteries type 1, and some strains of Shigella flexneri and Shigella sonnei excrete a toxin which is enterotoxin, neurotoxic and cytotoxic.

Question 22 Describe the symptoms of tuberculous meningitis.

Symptoms of Tuberculous Meningitis. The onset of the symptoms can be gradual. In children, the symptoms may present as lassitude, loss of interest in the surrounding, unwillingness to play,loss of appetite, headache, and constipation. In adults, the symptoms may be lethargy, headache, vomiting, and low-grade fever. In addition, both children and adults can have more severe symptoms like convulsions and **coma.**

Question 23 Discuss the role of lumbar puncture in patients with purulent meningitis.

Lumbar puncture is a diagnostic technique used in patients with purulent meningitis, which involves the removal of cerebrospinal fluid (CSF) for examination, measurement, and observationof the pressure in the CSF. The color of the CSF is purulent (turbid) due to the presence of neutrophils (> 1000 cells/ cubic mm), the pressure of the CSF will be increased, the protein content will be significantly increased, and the glucose will be reduced. Gram staining film and culture may reveal the causative organism, but the findings may be negative if the patients were treated earlier with antibiotics before the lumbar puncture examination. If the causative is known, then the antibiotics of choice, given intravenously depending on the age and weight of the patient, can be used effectively. A dull or throbbing headache is a frequent sequel of a lumbar puncture and may last for a few days. It is aggravated by erect posture and relieved with recumbency. It is due to leakage of the CSF through the dural puncture site. It may be prevented by using a smaller bored needle for the procedure and if the patient lies supine after the procedure for at least 6 hours.

References:

1. Harrison's Principle of Internal Medicine - 13th Edition.

2. Davidson's Principle and Practice of Medicine - 17th Edition,

Question 24 What diseases are caused by (1) adenovirus, *(2)* ECHO viruses, (3) Coxsackie viruses,and (4) respiratory syncytial viruses?

Diseases caused by Adenovirus are a Common cold with rhinitis, pharyngitis, and malaise without fever b. Acute non-streptococcal exudative pharyngitis c. Pharyngoconjunctival fever d.Acute keratoconjunctivitis e. Acute hemorrhagic cystitis f. Acute gastroenteritis.

Diseases caused by ECHO viruses are a. Aseptic meningitis b. Boston exanthem. c. Epidermis diarrhea. Common respiratory infections f. Myocarditis.

Diseases caused by Coxsackie viruses are a. Summer grippe (A and B) b. Herpangina (A2-6,10) c. Epidemic pleurodynia (B1-5) d. Aseptic meningitis. Acute nonspecific pericarditis f. Myocarditis (B1-5) g. Hand, foot, and mouth disease (A5, 10, 16)

Diseases caused by Respiratory Syncytial Viruses are a. Pneumonia b. Bronchiolitis c. Tracheobronchitis

References:

1. Harrison's Principles of Internal Medicine - 13th Edition.

2. Davidson's Principles and Practices of Medicine - 17th Edition.

Question 25 Discuss the treatment and prognosis of infectious mononucleosis.

Treatment of infectious mononucleosis

There is no specific treatment, and acyclic antiviral medications are not useful. The patient wouldneed symptomatic treatment and reassurance as the lethargy and lassitude may last for 2 to 3 months. Symptomatic treatment involves the use of aspirin and other non-steroidal anti-inflammatory drugs and warm saline gargles as required. Two days of corticosteroids (Hydrocortisone intravenously, 200 mg 6 hourly or Prednisolone orally, 10 mg 6 hourly) in patients with severe tonsillar swelling, which causes difficulty in swallowing and breathing. Steroids may be used in severe thrombocytopenia and autoimmune hemolytic anemia. However, steroids should not be used in uncomplicated acute infectious mononucleosis.

Prognosis of infectious mononucleosis

Fever may disappear in 10 days, and lymphadenopathy and splenomegaly in 4 weeks in uncomplicated cases. Feeling of lethargy and lassitude may last for 2 to 3 months. Most of the patients recover fully without serious complications. Some of the complications are myalgia encephalitis (chronic fatigue syndrome) which is common, and hepatitis, hemolytic anemia, thrombocytopenia, splenic rupture, and encephalitis rarely occur. Death is uncommon, andif it occurs, it is usually due to splenic rupture, severe hemolytic anemia, severe thrombocytopenic purpura, and encephalitis.

Question 26 What are the complications and sequelae of pertussis (whooping cough)?

Complications of Pertussis: a. Bronchitis b. Lobar pneumonia c. Atelectasis d. Conjunctival Hemorrhage. Ulceration of the frenulum f. Rectal prolapse g. Convulsion due to cerebral anoxia

Sequelae of Pertussis: Bronchiectasis.References:

1. Harrison's Principles of Internal Medicine - 13th Edition.
2. Davidson's Principles and Practices of Medicine - 17th Edition.

Question 27 Define epidemic parotitis (mumps). What complications may arise in the course of this disease?

Epidemic parotitis (mumps)

Epidemic parotitis (mumps) is an infection due to a paramyxovirus. It is spread by droplet infection, by direct contact, or through fomites. Humans are the only known natural hosts. The peak infectivity period is 2 to 3 days before the onset of the parotitis and to 3 days afterward.

Complications of epidemic parotitis (mumps). a. Meningitis b. Orchitis, and rarely priapism ortesticular infarction. c. Pancreatitis d. Oophoritis e. Thyroiditis f. Neuritis g. Myocarditis h.
Thrombocytopenic purpura I. Migratory arthralgias j. Nephritis k. Rare neurological complications- encephalitis, Guillain-Barre syndrome, transverse myelitis, and deafness due to8th nerve neuritis.

References:

1. Harrison's Principles of Internal Medicine - 13th Edition.

2. Davidson's Principles and Practices of Medicine - 17th Edition.

Question 28Discuss the various factors concerned with the common cold.

Common cold (acute coryza)

The common cold is the most common of all the viral causes of upper respiratory tract infections. It is usual for a person to have an attack of the common cold about 2 to 3 times a year. The infection is spread by close contact with the nasal mucus in the hands or by droplets, and it can be facilitated by poor ventilation and overcrowding. The incubation period is 12 hours to 5 days. The causative viruses are Rhinoviruses, coronaviruses, enteroviruses, adenoviruses, and respiratory syncytial viruses.

Clinical features:

The onset is rapid with sneezing, blocked nose, sore nose, and watery nasal discharge, which is clear and can be yellowish green after 24 to 48 hours in secondary bacterial infection. The patient maybe lethargic and have a headache, mild fever, and sore throat. The nasal examination may show a congested, edematous nasal mucosa and discharge.

Investigations.

Most of the patients will recover rapidly. Thus, investigations are done only for more severe illnesses. Viruses can be isolated from the exfoliated cells with throat swabs and identified with serological tests like fluorescent antibody tests. A culture of the throat swabs may be necessary to identify secondary bacterial infections. Radiography for chronic sinusitis may be needed forsome patients.

Treatment

Most of the patients will not require treatment. However, symptomatic treatment like antipyretics to relievefever and nasal decongestants like oxymetazoline and pseudoephedrine 30 mg every 4 hours or 120 mg twice a day for a few days may relieve nasal congestion and obstruction can be used.
Chronic use of nasal sprays may result in rhinitis medicamentosa, and it is treated with the complete withdrawal of nasal sprays, and a topical intranasal corticosteroid (flunisolide) or a short courseof oral steroids may be useful. Antibiotics are only used if there is a presence of secondary bacterial infection,

Complications.

1. Sinusitis 2. Pneumonia or bronchitis 3. Otitis media and hearing impairment due to theblockage of Eustachian tubes.

References:

1. Harrison's Principles of Internal Medicine - 13th Edition.
2. Davidson's Principles and Practices of Medicine - 17th Edition.

Question 29 List the prognostic factors in epidemic hemorrhagic fever (Manchurian Fever).

Prognostic factors in epidemic hemorrhagic fever are: The caustic organism is due to Hantaviruses which are enzootic viruses of wild rodents spread by aerosolized excretaand not by insect vectors. The poor prognostic signs are associated with renal involvement resulting in hemorrhagic fever with a renal syndrome, which carries a mortality rate of 5 to 10% and is characterized by fever, shock, and hemorrhage followed by an oliguric phase. The oliguric phase may lead to acute renal failure due to acute hemorrhagic interstitial nephritis. If untreated,the mortality is high, but the patient should recover with the proper treatment of acute renal failure and blood transfusion if necessary.

Question 30 What is the Stevens-Johnson Syndrome?

Stevens-Johnson Syndrome is a severe bullous erythema multiforme involving the mucosal in the mouth, eyes, and genitals, and toxic constitutional symptoms. It is also known as erythemamultiforme major. This syndrome is associated with drugs commonly like sulfonamides, non-steroidal anti-inflammatory drugs such as fenoprofen, and anticonvulsants such as phenytoin, barbiturates, and penicillamine and sulindac. It appears to be a target-like lesion and is found distributed mainly on the extensor aspects of the limbs. The lesions may show pallor accompanied by central erythema or purpura. The bullae represent epidermal necrosis and the separation of this layer. Mucous membrane ulcerations are frequent and painful during eating,swallowing, and urination.

Treatment.

Patients with extensive denudation of the skin are best treated in the burn unit. There is no specific treatment for Stevens-Johnson syndrome. Immediate cessation of the offending drug isimportant and supportive treatment, such as hydration, is also important. Corticosteroids are commonly given to patients, but there is no supporting data for their use.

Complications. Complications of the visceral lesions such as pneumonitis, myocarditis, nephritis, and scarring of tracheobronchial mucosa and conjunctiva.

References:

1. Harrison's Principle of Internal Medicine - 13th Edition,
2. Davidson's Principles and Practices of Medicine - 17th Edition.

Question 31 Define cat-scratch disease and its treatment.

Cat-scratch disease.

This acute infection occurs in children and young adults who are in contact with catsor dogs. A scratch or bite can transmit it. It is caused by Gram-negative bacillus Bartonella henselae or Rochalimaea henselae (formerly known). A small papule appears at the site between 7 to 14 days after a scratch or bite and is associated with regional lymphadenopathy, which persists for a few weeks and maybe suppurate. The disease may progress systematically withencephalitis, neuroretina, arthritis, hepatitis, osteolytic bone lesions, and pleurisy. An excisional biopsy of the lymph node with its characteristic pattern is diagnostic.

Treatment.

Symptoms usually resolve without specific therapy in 1 to 2 weeks. Antibiotics may not be necessary in uncomplicated cases. The organism is sensitive to some cephalosporins (cefoxitin,cefotaxime) and aminoglycosides (gentamicin, tobramycin) which can be used in complicated cases.

Question 32 Give the period of incubation and of the eruption of the exanthemata.

The period of incubation of exanthemata is 5 to 15 days.

The period of the eruption of exanthemata is on the fourth or fifth day of the illness when the rash appears suddenly, and the rash usually lasts for a few hours to 1 to 2 days. The rash is a faint 2 to3 mm macules or maculopapular over the neck, trunk, thighs, and buttocks.

Question 33 Give the symptoms of epidemic influenza,

Symptoms of epidemic influenza are:

The onset of the symptoms is abrupt, with fever which may last 1 to 7 days, chills, malaise,muscle aches, sternal tenderness, headache, nasal stuffiness and discharge, nausea, nonproductive cough, and sore throat.

References:

1. Harrison's Principles of Internal Medicine - 13th Edition,
2. Davidson's Principles and Practices of Medicine - 17th Edition.

Question 34 Give the etiology, symptoms, and treatment of acute anterior epidemic poliomyelitis.

Acute anterior epidemic poliomyelitis. A. Etiology. A susceptible person is infected with poliovirus 1, 2, or 3, a picorna virus, and it is usually spread by fecal-oral route as the virus is excreted in the feces. It tends to affect the central nervous system, especially the anteriorhorn cells of the spinal cord and the cranial nerve motor neurons. The incidence of poliomyelitisworldwide has decreased dramatically following the improvement of sanitation, hygiene, and the polio vaccine.

B. Symptoms. At least 95% of cases are asymptomatic, and the symptomatic cases are presented as a. Abortive poliomyelitis. It is characterized by fever, sore throat, headache, muscle aches, vomiting, diarrhea, and constipation. b. Nonparalytic poliomyelitis. All the above symptoms in abortive poliomyelitis and signs of meningeal irritation, but recovery is complete. c. Paralytic poliomyelitis. All the above symptoms of abortive poliomyelitis and signs of spinal poliomyelitisand bulbar poliomyelitis.

C. Treatment a. Strictly bed rest in the 'polio bed with frequent changing of position in the first few days of illness may reduce the rate of paralysis. b. Symptomatic treatment for the abortive poliomyelitis phase.

Question 35 Discuss the management of acute infectious hepatitis (virus A).

Management of acute infectious hepatitis (virus A).

a. Bed rest in the initial acute phase of the disease when the symptoms are most **severe.**

b. Immediate protection can be given by immune serum globulin soon after exposure to the virus, especially the persons at high risk, such as close contact, the elderly, pregnant women, and those with major diseases.

c. An infected person can excrete the virus in feces for about 2 to 6 weeks before the onset of theillness and for 5 to 7 days thereafter. Therefore, the infected person must be educated to avoid spreading the virus by fecal-oral route, especially via homosexual activity in men. In addition, this transient viremia in the incubation period may allow the infection to spread via blood.

d. Corticosteroids have no benefits, and admission to the hospital is usually not necessary. If the patient has severe nausea and vomiting, admission may_be considered for supportive treatment, likeintravenous administration of 10% glucose solution.

References:

1. Harrison's Principles of Internal Medicine - 13th Edition.
2. Davidson's Principles and Practices of Medicine - 17th Edition.

Question 36 What complications may occur with herpes zoster (shingles)?

The complications which may occur with herpes zoster are:

a. Secondary bacterial infection.

b. Post-herpetic neuralgia over the face or trunk may be intractable, especially in the elderly over the age of 60 years and in immunocompromised persons with malignant diseaseor ADS.

c. Trophic ulcers over the face in association with cranial nerve involvement.

d. Zoster ophthalmicus due to the involvement of the ophthalmic branch of the trigeminal nervewith eye infection, eyelid swelling, conjunctivitis, vesicles on the cornea with corneal ulceration, or blistering of the side of the nose.

e, Persistent anesthesia or scarring of the affected face or trunk following healing with facial oranother nerve paralysis.

f. Encephalitis and myelitis if the virus invades the brain or the spinal cord, respectively.

g. Segmental muscle wasting may occur from the involvement of the motor root.

h. Ramsay-Hunt syndrome is the herpes zoster infection of the geniculate ganglion that presents withvesicles in the auricle and on the palate, and the facial nerve involvement leads to ipsilateral facial paralysis and impairment of the taste.

References:

1. Harrison's Principles of Internal Medicine - 13th Edition,
2. Davidson's Principles and Practices of Medicine - 17th Edition.

Question 37 Differentially diagnose chancre, chancroid and herpes progenitalis.

Chancre. It is caused by Treponema pallidum, transmitted by sexual contact for both sexes.

Clinical features:

This lesion is found in primary syphilis, and it starts as a small erosion 3 to 4 weeks after inoculation that rapidly develops into a painless superficial ulcer with a clean base and firm, indurated margins with enlargement of the regional lymph nodes, which is rubbery, discrete, andnon-tender. The chancre may be painful if there is a bacterial infection and scarring on healing.

Investigations:

Serologic test for syphilis is usually positive 1 to 2

weeks after the primary lesion is noted. Immunofluorescence or darkfield microscopy shows treponemes in about 95% of the chances.

Chancroid. It is caused by a Gram-negative bacillus Hemophilus ducreyi, transmitted by sexual contact in both sexes, and nonvenereal inoculation has been reported in medical personnel.

Clinical features: The lesion starts as a vesicopustule that breaks down to form a painful, soft ulcer with a necrotic base, surrounding erythema, and undermined edges. The lesion is contagious and spreads to other sites. The inguinal lymph nodes are enlarged, tender, and matted withoverlying erythema, which may rupture spontaneously. Investigations: Culture of the swab from the lesions on chocolate agar with 1% Isovitalex and vancomycin, 3 mg/ml to show the Hemophilus ducreyi.

Herpes progenitalis. It is caused by Herpes simplex type 2 and is transmitted by sexualcontact for both sexes.

Clinical features.

There is a burning and stinging sensation with the eruption of small vesicles, most often on the lips, mouth, and buttocks. The vesicles will eventually crust and become non-infectious when allthe crusts fall off. The regional lymph nodes may become swollen and tender. It may cause painful perianal ulcerations in patients with AIDS. Investigations: Direct immunofluorescent antibody slide tests can offer a rapid diagnosis. Viral culture is helpful in confirming the clinical diagnosis.

References:

1. Harrison's Principles of Internal Medicine - 13th Edition.

2. Davidson's Principles and Practices of Medicine - 17th Edition.

Question 38 Differentiate the early eruption of syphilis and measles.

The early eruption of Syphilis occurs in the secondary stage of syphilis which happens about a few weeks to 6 months after the appearance of the chancre. The lesions on the skin are non-pruritic,macular, popular, pustular, or follicular; the most common is the maculopapular rash. The skin lesions are generalized and may involve the soles and palms. The lesions on the mucosa could be papules to ulcers on the lips, mouth, throat, genitalia, and anus and sometimes diffuse redness of the pharynx. In addition, there may have condylomata which are papules on the moist areas of the skin and mucosa membranes. These skin and mucosa lesions are highly contagious.

The early eruption of Measles is the Kolpik's spots that appear 2 days before the rash and willlast from 1 to 4 days as tiny white spots on the oral mucosa membrane and sometimes on the conjunctival folds vaginal mucous membrane. The rash will appear first on the face and behind the ears 4 days after the onset of the symptoms. The rashes appear as papules that coalesce to form a maculopapular rash. Then the rash next appears on the trunk and later on the extremities, palm and soles. The rash will fade away in the order of appearance.

Question 39 List the more common manifestations of congenital syphilis.

The common manifestations of congenital syphilis are:

<u>Early findings</u>: a. Stillbirth or failure to thrive b. Lesions on the skin and mucous membranes areSerous nasal discharge

with nasal infection - snuffles. Mucous membrane patches. Maculopapular rash Condylomas c. May have hepatosplenomegaly, anemia or osteochondritis.

Late findings: a. Stigmata of syphilis: Hutchinson's teeth, Sabre shins, saddle nose, and abnormalities of long bones. b. Others: interstitial keratitis, uveitis, facial gummas, deafness, andcentral nervous **system.**

References:

1. Harrison's Principles of Internal Medicine - 13th Edition.

2. Davidson's Principles and Practices of Medicine - 17th Edition.

Question 40 What does the term " making of syphilis " means?

"Making of syphilis" means experimental inoculation of treponema pallidum organisms of small numbers into rabbits or humans to produce the infection of syphilis. Intradermal injection of 100 organisms usually produces a lesion in about 72 hours. However, experimental inoculations of humans and rabbits show that from the time of the inoculation to the production ofthe primary lesion is about 6 weeks. The number of organisms required to produce the symptomsof syphilis was determined by the intradermal injection of graded doses of the organism simultaneously at separate sites.

Question 41 What is the treatment of choice for primary and secondary syphilis?

Treatment of choice for primary syphilis is Benzathine penicillin G, 2.4 million units intramuscularly in the gluteal region, single dose or Procaine penicillin, 600-1200 mg intramuscularly once a day for 2 weeks with probenecid,

500 mg orally four times a day for 2 weeks. For patients who are allergic to penicillin, doxycycline, 100 mg orally twice a day for 2weeks, or tetracycline, 500 mg orally four times a day for 2 weeks, can be used and provided that the female patient is not pregnant (erythromycin may be used here).

Treatment of choice of secondary syphilis is Treatment as above if there is no central nervous system (CNS) involvement. If the CNS is involved, then aqueous crystalline penicillin G, 2-4 million units intravenously every 4 hours for 2 weeks, or procaine penicillin, 2-4 million units intramuscularly in the gluteal region once a day with probenecid, 500 mg orally four times a dayfor 2 weeks. Alternatively, for patients who are allergic to penicillin, tetracycline, 500 mg orally four times a day for 3 weeks, or doxycycline, 100 mg orally twice a day for 3 weeks.

Question 42 What factors tend to influence the relapse rate of syphilis?

Factors that influence the relapse rate of syphilis are:

a. Secondary syphilis may relapse if undiagnosed.
b. Secondary syphilis may relapse if untreated inadequately.

Question 43 Is it advisable in treating neurosyphilis to administer bismuth or mercury before giving penicillin to avoid a possible Herxheimer reaction?

No it is not advisable.

References.

1. Harrison's Principles of Internal Medicine - 13th Edition,
2. Davidson's Principles and Practices of Medicine - 17th Edition.

Question 44 What represents the most important single cause of death in endemic typhus fever?

The most important single cause of death in endemic typhus fever is a circulatory failure, renal failure, or intercurrent bacterial infection.

Question 45 Differentiate clinically between endemic typhus and Rocky Mountain spotted fever.

Endemic Typhus	**Rocky Mountain spotted fever**
a. Incubation period 8 to 16 days	3 to 10 days
b. Symptoms Chills, rigors, fever, severe frontal headache, malaise, nausea, and vomiting. Frontal headaches may dominate the clinical picture and may have delirium, severe agitation, or coma. Conjunctival congestion is less common.	Fever, chills, headache, aches in bones, joints,muscles, and abdominal pain, nausea, vomiting, restlessness, irritability, insomnia, delirium, convulsions, coma. Flushed face and conjunctival congestion.
c. Signs Rash persists for 4 to 8 days. Generalized Muscular Rash progress to shoulders, chest, arms, and thighs. The sparse rash is seen over the face, palms, and soles., Macular rash which becomes maculopapular. Nonproductive irritating cough withbasilar rales. Accelerated pulse with	The rash persists for 2 to 3 days. Macular rash progress to maculopapular, then petechiae. The rash starts on the ankles and wrists, spreading centrally to the arms, legs, and trunk. Cough and pneumonitis may occur. Less often with accelerated pulse and hypotension. May have splenomegaly,

hypotension. Abdominal pain with diarrhea. Splenomegaly in 25% of cases.Hepatomegaly and jaundice areuncommon,	hepatomegaly, jaundice, gangrene, myocarditis, or uremia

References:

1. Harrison's Principles of Internal Medicine - 13th Edition.

2. Davidson's Principles and Practices of Medicine - 17th Edition.

Question 46 What is the chief clinical manifestation of psittacosis (ornithosis)?

Chief clinical manifestations of psittacosis (ornithosis are: Symptoms: Malaise, high-graded fever, cough, and muscular pain. Sometimes may present as high swinging fever, photophobia, and neck stiffness.

Signs: Scanty pinkish-red "rose spots" over the abdomen and hepatosplenomegaly.

Question 47 Give the clinical picture of an untreated lymphogranuloma venereum (lymphopathia venereum climatic bubo).

The clinical picture of an untreated case of lymphogranuloma venereum is as follows: The first primary lesion is a painless ulcerating papule on the genitalia, which will heal in a few days with the development of regional lymphadenopathy. The lymph nodes are painful and fixed, and the overlyingskin will develop a dusky erythematous appearance. Later, the lymph nodes will become fluctuant (buboes) and may rupture. Sometimes, the patient may present with proctitis and perirectal abscesses.

Question 48 Describe the clinical features of coccidioidomycosis.

The clinical features of coccidioidomycosis are: Many of the patients are asymptomatic. After an incubation of 10 days, the patients may present with acute pulmonary coccidioidomycosis with fever, malaise, cough, and expectoration. Although erythema nodosum, erythema multiforme, phlyctenularconjunctivitis, and pleural effusions may occur, the patient mostly fully recovers. Patients with more severe forms of coccidioidomycosis may develop pulmonary cavitation with hemoptysis, pulmonary fibrosis, meningitis, lytic bone lesions, hepatosplenomegaly, skin abscesses, and skin ulcers.

References:

1. Harrison's Principles of Internal Medicine - 13th Edition.
2. Davidson's Principles and Practices of Medicine - 17th Edition.

Question 49 Discuss the symptomatology of toxoplasmosis.

The symptomatology of toxoplasmosis is: The commonest presentation is asymptomatic lymphadenopathy. The lymphadenopathy is associated with acute febrile illness and cervical lymph node involvement. In the acute febrile infection, there may be fever, malaise,sore throat, headache, myalgia, arthralgia, and jaundice with maculopapular rash, hepatosplenomegaly, uveitis, chorioretinitis, myocarditis, and hepatitis. The symptomatic neurological presentation may be a headache, neck stiffness, and confusion. In congenital toxoplasmosis, the patients may present with headache, confusion, and the characteristic "Syndrome of Savin," which is internal encephala's, chorioretinitis, convulsions, and cerebral calcifications, tremors, nystagmus, microphthalmia, and pneumonitis may be present. The surviving patients will exhibit symptoms of mental retardation, epilepsy, and spastic paraplegia.

Question 50 Discuss the problems concerned with the treatment of histoplasmosis.

The problems concerned with the treatment of histoplasmosis are: The usual drug used is itraconazole which is used in patients with severe and progressive localized disease and nonmeningeal disseminated disease of histoplasmosis. Amphotericin B is used for patients who are unable to tolerate it orally, failure of itraconazole treatment, patients with meningitis, or patientswith disseminated disease in immunocompromised patients. Amphotericin B has many toxic side effects like anorexia, nausea, fever, headache, venous thrombosis, and renal toxicity.

The venous thrombosis can be controlled by adding prednisolone with Amphotericin Btreatment. Plasma urea and creatinine must be monitored for renal toxicity, which is common in patients who require Amphotericin B for a long period.

Question 51 Define and give treatment for actinomycosis.

Definition of actinomycosis:

Actinomycosis is caused by actinomyces israelii, an anaerobic commensal in the mouth, which isa bacterial infection and not a fungal infection. Actinomycosis may cause cervicofacial, abdominal, and pulmonary infection with suppurative pneumonia, empyema, and chest wall sinuses. In addition, the pus may contain "Sulphur grains."

Treatment of Actinomycosis

The drug of choice is benzylpenicillin 2 to 4 grams intravenously every 6 hours for 4 to 6 weeksand followed by oral penicillin for a couple of weeks after clinical resolution. If the patient is allergic to penicillin, then he may use tetracycline. Treatment may sometimes involve surgery.

References:

1. Harrison's Principles of Internal Medicine - 13th Edition.
2. Davidson's Principles and Practices of Medicine - 17th Edition.

Question 52 Give two types of nocardiosis and their treatment.

The two types of nocardiosis are:

1. Pulmonary nocardiosis: The patient may present with cough, fever, loss of weight, night sweats and hemoptysis. Pleural involvement and empyema may occur in the patient.

2. Systemic nocardiosis: The dissemination of nocardiosis may involve any organ, especiallybrain abscesses, and also a local invasion of the subcutaneous tissue. Mycetoma is the local invasion by Nocardia on, usually, the sole of the foot, as a painless swelling (Madura's foot).
Nodules may appear from the purulent fluid containing "grains" of

the organisms are discharged

Treatment of nocardiosis: Treatment consists of adequate surgical drainage of the pus combinedwith chemotherapy. Chemotherapy was initiated with intravenous trimethoprim-sulfamethoxazole and continued with oral trimethoprim-sulfamethoxazole, one double-strength tablet twice a day.

Question 53 Give the symptoms related to the three periods of development in trichinosis.

The symptoms related to the three periods of development in trichinosis are:

1. First 24 to 72 hours after ingestion of the contaminated meat with Trichinella spiralis, thepatient may present with vomiting, diarrhea, abdominal pain, and headache.

2. The second week to 1 to 2 months, the patient may present with muscle pain and tenderness, muscle spasms, fever, periorbital and facial edema, conjunctivitis, and photophobia. An urticaria rash, diarrhea, dyspnea, and pleurisy may occur.

3. In the third stage, the larvae encyst in the striated muscle and may cause weakness, musclepain, and cramps, which may persist for several months.

Question 54 List the complications of bacillary dysentery.

Complications of bacillary dysentery are:

1. Mild complications: arthritis, conjunctivitis, morbilliform rash, temporary disaccharidase deficiency following diarrhea, and uncommonly,

Reiter's syndrome.

2. Severe complications: colonic perforation, septicemia, and hemolytic uremic syndrome withrenal failure.

References:

1. Harrison's Principles of Internal Medicine - 13th Edition.
2. Davidson's Principles and Practices of Medicine - 17th Edition.

Question 55 Give the symptomatology and complications of amebiasis.

Symptoms of amebiasis:

A. Intestinal manifestations:

1. Gradual onset: the patient may have mild intermittent diarrhea and abdominal pain, weight loss, fatigue, and progressing to bloody diarrhea with mucus. General symptoms like headache, nausea and anorexia may be present.

2. Severe acute colitis: patients become more toxic with high-graded fever, vomiting, abdominal colic and tenderness, and a non-specific hepatic enlargement and tenderness.

3. Fulminating colitis: patient appears very unwell with low-graded fever, which may be absent.There might be hypotension, paralytic ileus, massive mucosal sloughing, and hemorrhage.

B. Extraintestinal manifestations:

1. Hepatic amebiasis: patient will high graded fever, abdominal pain over the right hypochondrium, and a tender enlarged liver. There may also be sweating, chills,

anorexia, weightloss, and malaise.

2. Skin infections over the perianal region. Metastatic infection to the lungs, brain, and genitalia is commonly.

Complications of amebiasis are:

1. Progression of the fulminant colitis to toxic dilatation of the colon with perforation and peritonitis, peri colonic abscess, retroperitoneal fecal cellulitis, and fistula to the abdominalsurface.
2. Chronic infection leads to stricture formation.
3. Severe hemorrhage.
4. Ameboma is the mass of fibrotic granulation tissue in the caecum or rectosigmoid region. It may bleed and cause obstruction and intussusception.
5. Amebic liver abscess, which may occur without the stage of colitis.
6. Appendicitis.

References:

1. Harrison's Principles of Internal Medicine - 13th Edition,

2. Davidson's Principles and Practices of Medicine - 17th Edition.

Question 56 Discuss the clinical manifestations and treatment of moniliasis (candida albicans infection).

Clinical manifestations of moniliasis. Moniliasis is a superficial infection of the skin, nails, and mucous membrane. Skin infections occur typically in the intertriginous areas where they are moist, like in the groins, perineum, breasts, and axillae. This cutaneous moniliasis can bevery pruritic. Nail infections start at the nail's base and form ridges and paronychia. In the mouth, the white curd-like patch can be scraped, causing a bleeding base, atrophy of the gums, and angular stomatitis are common in elderly patients. Vaginitis cause intense pruritus and a thick, smelly discharge. In children, cutaneous moniliasis can cause widespread involvement of the skin, nails, hair, and mucosae, which may respond poorly to treatment. Systemic moniliasis may cause septicemia and features of the infection of the gastrointestinaltract, the esophagus, heart, lungs, urinary tract, and in the meningeal layers of the brain,

Treatment of moniliasis. The first thing is to control and treat the predisposition cause of the moniliasis. Cutaneous moniliasis can be treated with topical azole ointment. Oral moniliasis respond well to oral nystatin, oral amphotericin or miconazole. Persistent infections may need oral ketoconazole or itraconazole 100 mg daily for a few months. Vaginal moniliasis can be treatedwith pessaries or cream containing one of the imidazole antifungals, such as clotrimazole, used intravaginally. Nystatin can also be used. If the topical treatment fails, triazole drugs such as fluconazole 150 mg single dose or itraconazole 200 mg twice a day may be used systemically. The male partner of the woman should be reviewed and possibly treated. For any severe systemic infection, intravenous treatment with amphotericin, ketoconazole, or flucytosine 50-75 mg/kg daily for 2 to 3 weeks may be needed.

References.

1. Harrison's Principles of Internal Medicine - 13th Edition.
2. Davidson's Principles and Practices of Medicine - 17th Edition.

Question 57 Discuss the chemotherapy for malaria.

Chemotherapy of Malaria.

A. Supportive and general treatment. Patients may be given analgesics and antipyretics. Intravenous fluids may need to treat dehydration and shock.

B. Treatment of an acute attack of malaria. The drug of choice is 4-aminoquinolones. Chloroquine-sensitive malaria is treated with chloroquine 600 mg as the loading dose and followed by 300 mg in 6 hours and then 150 mg twice daily for 3 days, or amodiaquine hydrochloride 600mg loading dose followed by 400 to 600 mg daily for two days up to a maximum dose of 2400 mg. Patients with chloroquine-resistant malaria should be treated quinine sulfate 650 mg three times a day for 5 days, given in combination with pyrimethamine 25 mg twice daily for 3 days and sulphadiazine 500 mg twice daily for 5 days. Mefloquine and halofantrine can also be used to treat resistant malaria cases.

C. Treatment of severe malaria. Severe malaria is a medical emergency as more than 1% of theRBC infected or any pernicious forms of malaria. The drug of choice here is quinine, given by slow intravenous infusion, Quinine dihydrochloride 20 mg/kg intravenously over 4 hours followed by 100 mg/kg infusion over 4 hours at 8 hourly intervals until the patient can tolerate oral therapy.

D. Specific treatments.

1. Plasmodium falciparum. Chloroquine alone or combined with either pyrimethamine 25mg or primaquine 45 mg as a single dose can result in a radical cure as there is no exoerythrocytic stage in falciparum malaria.

2. P. vivax, P malariae, Povale. Primaquine is used to eradicate the exoerythrocytic stage for a radical cure. A course of one of the 4-aminoquinolones should be followed by primaquine 7.5 mg daily for 14 days. Alternatively, 300 mg chloroquine combined with 45 mg primaquine oncea week for 8 weeks is also effective.

Question 58 Outline the management of the inflammatory stage of dermatophytosis (athletic foot, trichopytosis).

The drying effect of the foot powders, which contain antifungal agents of low potency, may be useful if applied regularly. Potassium permanganate 0.01% solution is a useful dry foot soak that canprevent maceration of the inflamed foot and prevent infection. Together with the above treatment, the patient should be given griseofulvin orally for up to 3 months of 500 mg twice a day for Trichophyton rubrum. Patients should also use clotrimazole or miconazole applied as a cream at night and as talc powder during the day.

References.

1. Harrison's Principles of Internal Medicine - 13th Edition,
2. Davidson's Principles and Practices of Medicine - 17th Edition.

Question 59 Outline the causes of allergy.

The causes of allergy.

A. Inhalants, Pollens, mold spores, animal waste (urine, saliva, dung), house dust mites, insects,drugs, airborne organic dusts, microorganisms, and organic chemicals.

B. Injections. Foods and drugs.

C. Injections. Drugs, Hymenoptera venom, and injected atopic allergens.

D. Contactants. Plants oil, cosmetics, perfumes, nickel in jewelry and on the buckles, undergarment fasteners, hair dyes, topical medications, occupational chemicals, gloves, catheters, dental dams, and other medical devices.

Question 60 Of what value are elimination diets and provocative feedings?

Elimination diets. The elimination diet is a very effective treatment method for any food allergy.A patient allergic to one or more types of food should be very vigilant at parties or restaurants, as a minute amount of food may be fatal.

Provocative feedings. This is a valuable test for patients suspected of food allergy where a double-blind placebo-controlled oral challenge is done. If the reported clinical findingsare reproduced, then the patient is an allergy to that food. Freeze-dried food in large opaque capsules is used for the testing.

Question 61 Define asthma and name four types.

Definition of asthma. Asthma is a disease characterized by increased responsiveness of the trachea and bronchi to various stimuli and manifested by widespread narrowing of the airwaysthat changes in severity either spontaneously or as a result of treatment,

Types of asthma. 1. Exercise-induced asthma 2. Triad asthma is a combination of asthma, aspirinsensitivity, and nasal polyposis. 3. Occupational asthma 4. Drug-induced asthma.

References.

1. Harrison's Principles of Internal Medicine - 13th Edition.
2. Davidson's Principles and Practices of Medicine - 17th Edition.

Question 62 What are autoimmune diseases?

<u>Autoimmune diseases.</u> An autoimmune disease occurs when the immune system fails to recognize the body's tissues as "self" and mounts an attack on them. Autoimmune diseases can be divided into those that affect just one organ (organ-specific) and those which affect manysystems (organ non-specific or multi-systemic). Autoimmune diseases are mostly of unknown etiology, although genetic, hormonal, microbiological, and environmental factors are known to beimplicated in their manifestations and severity. Some examples are rheumatoid arthritis, thyroiditis, and pernicious anemia.

Question 63 Give the treatment of infective asthma.

<u>Treatment of infective asthma.</u> After the sputum Gram-staining and culture, an empirical courseof antibiotics is given. Amoxicillin or amoxicillin-potassium clavulanate, 500 mg orally every 8hours for 7 to 10 days, or tetracycline, 250-500 mg four times daily orally for 7 to 10 days, or trimethoprim-sulfamethoxazole, 160/800 mg orally every 12 hours for 7 to 10 days.
Supplemental oxygen, 1 to 3 L/min by nasal cannula, is given. Inhalation metered dose inhaler By-agonist drug like metaproterenol, 0.3 ml of 5% solution or albuterol, 0.5 ml of 0.5% solutiondiluted in 2,5 ml sterile normal saline using a powered nebulizer. Corticosteroids may be used orally or intravenously in severe asthma or if the patient fails to respond to the sympathomimetic therapy,

Question 64 Differentiate between urticaria, eczema, and angioneurotic edema.

Eczema.

Eczema is atopic dermatitis that is pruritic, exudative, or lichenified eruption on the face, neck, upper trunk, wrists and hands, and in the folds of knees and elbows. There may be a personal or a family history of atopic disease and a tendency to recur with remission from adolescence to age 20.

Urticaria and angioneurotic edema.

Urticaria is an intermittent transient swelling of the skin with fluid loss from the vessels intothe extravascular space. The lesions are itchy red swelling with wheals and erythema. The different forms of urticaria are dermographism, cholinergic urticaria, solar urticaria and cold urticaria. If there are a deeper vessel involvement, there may be swelling of the lips, tongue, eyelids, larynx, palms, soles, and genitalia, and this is called angioneurotic edema, which is serious and can be life-threatening.

References.

1. Harrison's Principles of Internal Medicine - 13th Edition.
2. Davidson's Principles and Practices of Medicine - 17th Edition.

Question 65 Discuss the clinical manifestations of stings of five Hymenoptera that occasionally cause death.

The clinical manifestations of the Hymenoptera's stings are: After the inoculation of the sting bythe hymenopterous insects, the patient will feel a sharp pain for several minutes, local wheal anderythema, and later, severe itching. The clinical signs of the insect bite will subside in a few hours. Unusual reactions such as optic neuritis, generalized polyneuropathy, myasthenia gravis, and acute renal failure due to venom-induced rhabdomyolysis and renal ischemia may be followingthe insect's sting. If a string is directly on a peripheral nerve, it may destroy the nerve function fora short period of time, like Bell's palsy if the sting is on the facial nerve. If the patient is hypersensitive to the sting, then the patient may show anaphylaxis with urticaria, nausea, abdominal or uterine cramps, bronchospasm, edema of the face and glottis, dyspnea, cyanosis, hypotension, coma, and sometimes death. Patients with previous experience of the sting with respiratory difficulty, hypotension, or generalized urticaria are in danger of a serious reaction if stung by the same insect again.

Question 66 Outline treatment of status asthmaticus.

The treatment of status asthmaticus. Care in the intensive care unit: 1. Controlled oxygen flow40-60%, given. 2. Nebulized albuterol 5 mg or terbutaline 10 mg is repeated and administered every 4 hours. 3. Intravenous hydrocortisone 200 mg is given 4 hourly for 24 hours. Prednisolone is continued at 60 mg orally for two weeks. 4. Antibiotics for presumed or provenairway infection. 5. Measure the PEFR to monitor the progress. 6. Arterial blood gases are measured. If the PaCon is more than 7 kPa, mechanical ventilation may be considered 7. Chest X-ray is performed to rule out pneumothorax. 8. Intravenous fluid is necessary to maintaina state of normal hydration, 9. If no improvement is seen, then intravenous infusion of albuterol 3-20 microgram/min or terbutaline 1.5-5 microgram/min is given 10. If the patient still progresses to respiratory acidemia, tracheal intubation and mechanical ventilation are warranted. 11. If the patient's condition is still not controlled, then an aggressive therapy of sedation with a benzodiazepine and general anesthesia with a Broncho was dilating anesthetic agents, like halothane andsegmental bronchial lavage to remove plugs of mucus may be necessary.

References.

1. Harrison's Principles of Internal Medicine - 13th Edition.
2. Davidson's Principles and Practices of Medicine - 17th Edition.

Question 67 Give the symptoms associated with acute systemic lupus erythematosus (SLE).

The symptoms associated with acute SLE.

A. General features. Malaise, tiredness, arthralgia, anorexia, and loss of weight.

B. The joints. Painful joints with or without active synovitis. There is seldom deforming arthritis.

There may be soft tissue swelling around the joints. Aseptic necrosis of the hip and knee is a rarecomplication.

C. The skin. Erythema with a butterfly distribution over the cheeks of the face and across the bridge of the nose. Vasculitis lesions on the fingertips and purpura and urticaria around the nail folds. Raynaud's phenomenon, livedo reticularis, palmar and plantar rashes, pigmentation, and alopecia may occur. Discoid lupus is a benign skin disease that occurs over the face and progresses to scarring and pigmentation.

D. The lungs. Clinical features of recurrent pleurisy, pleural effusions, pneumonitis, atelectasis, and pulmonary fibrosis may occur.

E. The heart. Pericarditis and myocarditis may occur with small pericardial effusions and cardiac failure resulting from myocarditis and hypertension. Aortic valve lesions, cardiomyopathy, and mitral valve endocarditis may rarely occur.

F. The kidneys. Proteinuria with minimal change, proliferating changes, or membranous: glomerulonephritis. Hypertension occurs due to nephrotic syndrome or renal failure.

G. The nervous system. Mild depression, epilepsy, cerebellar ataxia, aseptic meningitis, cranialnerve lesions, cerebrovascular accidents, or peripheral neuropathy.

H. The eyes. Conjunctivitis, photophobia,

transient blindness, blurring of vision.I.

The gastrointestinal system causes

Nausea, vomiting, anorexia, and diarrhea.

J. Other clinical features: arterial and venous thrombosis, lymphadenopathy, splenomegaly, Hashimoto's thyroiditis, hemolytic anemia, and thrombocytopenic purpura.

References.

1. Harrison's Principles of Internal Medicine - 13th Edition.

2. Davidson's Principles and Practices of Medicine - 17th Edition,

Question 68 Discuss the diagnosis and treatment of polyarteritis (periarteritis nodosa).

Diagnosis of polyarteritis nodosa (PAN). The diagnosis of PAN is based on clinical features and investigations. Clinical features of PAN. The initial features are non-specific, such as fever, malaise, severe weight, myalgia, and arthralgia. The later features are renal impairment, hypertension, polyneuropathy, lung disease, and cardiac problems, including arrhythmia, heart failure, and myocardial infarction. Migratory arthralgia or arthritis with fever is seen, and abdominal pain due to the liver and gastrointestinal tract involvement is common. Death can be dueto renal disease.

Investigation of PAN. The ESR is raised. The diagnosis depends on histological examination of the biopsy material from an affected organ or angiographic demonstration ofmicroaneurysms in hepatic, intestinal, or renal vessels.

Treatment of PAN, using corticosteroids in high doses, 60 mg of prednisolone daily, may control fever and other constitutional symptoms and heal vascular lesions. Combination treatment with immunosuppressive drugs, like azathioprine or cyclophosphamide, 2 mg/kg/daily,may improve the patient's survival. The dose of cyclophosphamide must be reduced in patients with renal failure.

Question 69 What is the significance of erythema nodosum?

The significance of erythema nodosum. Erythema nodosum is an immunological reaction that appears as acute or recurrent panniculitis that produces painful nodules or plaques on the shinsand may spread to the arms and thighs.

When this condition is noted, investigations need to be done to exclude the cause of erythema nodosum. The common causes of erythema nodosum are due to:

A. Drugs: Sulphonamides, oral contraceptive pill, penicillin, bromide.
B. Systemic diseases. Sarcoidosis, inflammatory bowel disease.
C. Infections. Bacteria and viruses: Streptococci, tuberculosis, leprosy, yersinia, cat scratchdisease. Chlamydia: psittacosis, lymphogranuloma venereum. Fungal: histoplasmosis, coccidiomycosis, blastomycosis.
D. Pregnancy.

References.

1. Harrison's Principles of Internal Medicine - 13th Edition.

2. Davidson's Principles and Practices of Medicine - 17th Edition.

Question 70 Describe the pulmonary and esophageal manifestations of progressive systemicsclerosis (scleroderma).

The pulmonary manifestations of scleroderma. The patient may have lower lobe fibrosis leadingto cyst formation and honeycombing in advanced cases. Gas transfer and restrictive ventilating defects are seen. Aspiration pneumonia and pulmonary hypertension may occur.

The esophageal manifestations of scleroderma. Most patients may have esophageal involvement with symptoms of heartburn or dysphagia. A barium swallow may show delayed peristalsis, dilatation, or stricture formation. Esophageal manometry is the most sensitive test.This test may show a lack of distal esophageal peristalsis and reduced esophageal sphincter pressure.

Question 71 Define chronic laryngitis and provide treatment for it.

Chronic laryngitis can be due to a few causes like

1. Repeated attacks of acute laryngitis. 2. Excessive use of voice. 3. Heavy smoking of tobacco.
4. Mouth breathing from nasal obstruction. 5. Chronic infection of the nasal sinuses.

The patient may present with hoarseness of voice, sometimes, the voice may be lost completely (aphonia). In addition, there will be irritation in the throat and spasmodic cough. In untreated,long-standing cases, the voice may be lost permanently.

Treatment.

The voice must be rested completely, especially for public speakers and teachers. Smoking mustbe stopped completely. Medicated steam inhalation may provide some relief.

References.

1. Harrison's Principles of Internal Medicine - 13th Edition.
2. Davidson's Principles and Practices of Medicine - 17th Edition.

Question 72 Discuss the value of bronchoscopy in diagnosis and treatment.

The value of flexible fiberoptic bronchoscopy in diagnosis and treatment. 1. Evaluation of the airway. 2. Diagnosis and staging of bronchogenic carcinoma. 3. Evaluation of hemoptysis. 4. Biopsy of lung infiltrates.

5. Diagnosis of pulmonary infections. 6. Facilitation of bronchoalveolar lavage. 7. Removal of retained secretions and foreign bodies from the airway.

The value of rigid bronchoscopy in diagnosis and treatment. 1. Massive bleeding. 2. Extractionof large obstructing objects, like foreign objects, blood clots, tumor masses, and broncholiths. 3. Biopsy of tracheal or main stem bronchus tumors and bronchial carcinoids. 4. Facilitation ofventilation during bronchoscopy. 5. Facilitation of laser therapy.

Question 73 Name the most common causes of hemoptysis.

Most common causes of hemoptysis. 1. Bronchial carcinoma. 2. Bronchiectasis. 3. Acute bronchitis. 4. Tuberculosis. 5. Suppurative pneumonia. 6. Pulmonary embolus and infarction. 7.Acute left ventricular failure. 8. Mitral stenosis.

Question 74 Differentiate hemoptysis and hematemesis.

Hemoptysis is the production of blood-stainedsputum.

Hematemesis is the vomiting of blood.

References.

1. Harrison's Principles of Internal medicine - 13thh Edition.
2. Davidson's Principles and Practices of Medicine - 17th Edition,

Question 75 Give causes and treatment for hemothorax.

Cause of hemothorax. Hemothorax is the presence of blood in the pleural space, usually due to atrauma to the chest.

Treatment of hemothorax. A very small hemothorax that is stable and improving on the chest X-ray may be managed without tube drainage. For large hemothorax, immediate insertion of a chest tube to control bleeding by the opposition of pleural spaces. As much blood as possible should be drained before the chest tube is removed. Thoracotomy may be necessary to control bleeding, remove large amounts of blood clots, and treat complications like bronchopleural fistula.

Question 76 Distinguish pleural effusion, pneumothorax, and atelectasis by physical examination.

	PLEURAL EFFUSION	***PEUNOMOTHROX***	**ATELECTASIS**
1. Chest movement	Reduced or absent on the affected side	Reduced or absent on the affected side	Reduced or absent on the affected side
2. Mediastinal shift	Towards the opposite side	Towards the opposite side	Towards Lesion
3. Percussion sound	Stony dull	Normal or Hyper-resonant	Dull
4. Breath sound	Decreased or absent	Decreased or absent	Decreased or absent
5. Vocal resonance	Decreased or absent	Decreased or absent	Decreased or absent
6. Added sound	Pleural rub above effusion	None	None

References.

1. Harrison's Principles of Internal Medicine - 13th Edition,
2. Davidson's Principles and Practices of Medicine - 17th Edition.

Question 77 List the causes of hemorrhagic pleural fluid. What are the recommended treatments?

Cause of hemorrhagic pleural fluids.

1. Trauma to the chest wall
2. Carcinoma of the bronchus
3. Pulmonary infarction
4. Pulmonary embolism

Recommended treatment.

Treatment is directed to the cause of the hemorrhagic pleural fluids 1. A small and stable hemorrhagic pleural fluid due to trauma may be managed without tube drainage. If there is a large hemorrhage, then immediate insertion of the chest tube is important to control the bleedingby opposing the pleural space. As much blood is drainage before the chest tube is removed. 2. Ifthe carcinoma of the bronchus is unresectable, then treatment is directed to the tumor by chemotherapy and radiotherapy. 3. Pulmonary embolism is managed with anticoagulants and thrombolytic therapy.

Question 78 Describe the management of pleurisy with effusion.

Management of pleurisy with effusion Aspiration of the pleural fluid may be necessary to relievethe breathlessness. It is not advisable to remove more than 1 liter on the first occasion, as pulmonary edema may occur following the aspiration of a large amount. A chest X-ray must be taken after the procedure as the complication of pneumothorax may occur. Treatment of the underlying causes, like pneumonia, heart failure, pulmonary embolism, and subphrenic abscess, is necessary for the complete resolution. Pleural effusions due to malignant infiltration may re-accumulate rapidly. Therefore, the pleural space can be obliterated with the injection of substances, like tetracycline, mustine hydrochloride, and inactivated Corynebacterium parvum into the space (pleurodesis) which produce an inflammatory reaction and extensive pleural adhesions.

References.

1. Harrison's Principles of Internal Medicine - 13th Edition.

2. Davidson's Principles and Practices of Medicine - 17th Edition.

Question 79 Differentiate chronic bronchitis and bronchiectasis.

	Chronic bronchitis.	Bronchiectasis
Definition	A productive cough with mucoid sputum for 3 months or more in each year	Dilatation of the bronchi withcopious purulent sputum
Causes	Cigarette smoking, Repeatedattacks of acute bronchitis. Chronic infection in the lowerand upper respiratory tract. Low-grade infection due toinefficiency of protective mechanisms, like pneumococci and H.influenzae	Infection due to bronchial obstruction caused by intraluminal foreign bodiesmucus, inflammatory exudates, pus, tumor orstricture of the wall, and pressure from outside the wall by enlarged lymph nodes, tumor invasions and tuberculosis. Sequalae t measles and whooping

		cough
Gross	Bronchi may be dilated, and mucous membrane thickenedwith mucous secretions.	Saccular dilatations of bronchi with inflamed walls.
Microscopic	Increase in mucous glands in submucosa with hyperplasia and chronic inflammatory cell infiltration	Bronchial wall infiltrated by chronic inflammatory tissue with fibrous replacement
Clinical Features	Wheezing, breathlessness with scanty mucoid sputum. Inspiratory and expiratory rhonchi with fine crepitations.	Chronic productive cough with purulent sputum in the morning. Coarse crepitationsin basal area.

Question 80 What is the treatment of bronchiectasis?

Treatment of bronchiectasis.

1. Postural drainage. Lying over the side of the bed with head and trunk down or bya physiotherapist at least three times a day for 10 to 20 minutes.

2. Antibiotics based on the sputum Gram-staining and cultures. If bacterial pathogens cannot beidentified, then empirical treatment with oral antibiotics for 10 to 14 days with amoxicillin- clavulanate, 500 mg every 8 hours, or ampicillin or tetracycline, 250 to 500 mg 4 times daily, or

trimethoprim-sulfamethoxazole, 160/800 mg every 12 hours for patients with an acute exacerbation. In patients with stable bronchiectasis and copious purulent sputum, alternating cycles of two or three of the above antibiotics can be given orally for 2 to 4 weeks.

3. Bronchoscopy may be used to evaluate hemoptysis, remove retained secretions, and rule outobstructing lesions.

4. Surgery is reserved for patients with localized bronchiectasis who do not respond to theabove treatment. Surgery is also indicated for massive hemoptysis.

References.

1. Harrison's Principles of Internal Medicine - 13th Edition.
2. Davidson's Principles and Practices of Medicine - 17th Edition.

Question 81 Describe the etiology of spontaneous pneumothorax and outline the management.

Etiology of spontaneous pneumothorax.

1. Primary pneumothorax. a. Traumatic b. Iatrogenic- after procedures like thoracentesis, pleuralbiopsy, subclavian line placement, percutaneous lung biopsy, bronchoscopy with transbronchial biopsy, positive-pressure mechanical ventilation.

2. Secondary pneumothorax as a complication of a Tuberculosis b. Asthma c. Chronicobstructive airway disease, d. Infiltrating lung diseases, like pneumocystis pneumonia.

Management of spontaneous pneumothorax. Treatment depends on the severity of pneumothoraxand the nature of the cause of it. The patient with a small new pneumothorax (<15%) should be admitted to the hospital for observation for 2 days and placed on bed rest, treated for the cough and chest pain, and followed by serial X-ray every 12-24 hours. The small pneumothorax may resolvespontaneously by itself. The small pneumothorax may progress to tension pneumothorax, or a patient with severely symptomatic or a large pneumothorax (>15%) must have a chest tube placement done immediately, which is then placed under water-sealed drainage, and suction is applied until the lungs expand. For tension pneumothorax, a large bored needle should be inserted immediately, and the chest tube insertion thereafter. Recurrent pneumothorax should be treated by obliteration of the pleural space by chemical pleurodesis, using kaolin, or by pleural abrasion or parietal pleurectomy at thoracotomy.

Treatment of the cause of secondary pneumothorax is important, like chemotherapy for tuberculosis. Patients must stop smoking as the recurrence is about 50%. Exposure to highaltitudes, flying in unpressurized aircraft, and scuba diving should be avoided.

Question 82 Outline the treatment of primary lung abscess.

Treatment of primary lung abscess. Anaerobic bacterial pathogens are found in up to 70% of lung abscesses, but there is usually a mixed flora with aerobic bacterial pathogens. Therefore, antibiotics should be given to cover both aerobic and anaerobic pathogens. Treatment should be cefuroxime 1 gram intravenously for 6 hourly, erythromycin, 500 mg intravenously 8 hourly, and metronidazole, 500 mg intravenously 8 hourly for 5 days, and treatment is continued, followed bythe bacterial culture sensitivity. Surgery may be needed to drain the lung abscess.

References.

1. Harrison's Principles of Internal Medicine - 13th Edition.

2. Davidson's Principles and Practices of Medicine - 17th Edition.

Question 83 What is the significance of calcified pulmonary nodules?

The significance of calcified pulmonary nodules is that the lesion is almost certainly benign.Conversely, malignant pulmonary nodules are rarely calcified.

Question 84 How would you diagnose carcinoma of the lungs?

Carcinoma of the lungs.

A. Chest X-ray. It is the most used screening test for carcinoma of the lungs. It is the relatively insensitive test as the tumor mass must be between 1 to 2 cm in size to be reliably recognized. The chest X-ray can demonstrate up to 90% of the carcinoma during clinical presentation.Lung carcinoma can appear as round shadows on the chest X-ray. Sometimes, the edge of the tumor has a fluffy or spiked appearance.

B. Computed tomography. CT is useful identifying of pathological changes in the mediastinum and identifying the secondary spread of carcinoma to the opposite lung by detectingmasses too small to be seen by chest X-ray.

C. Fiberoptic bronchoscopy. It is used to obtain cytological specimens from the peripherallesions and biopsy evidence of any tumors seen.

D. Transthoracic fine-needle aspiration biopsy. This involves the direct aspiration through the chest wall of peripheral lung lesions under X-ray and CT screening. Specimens can be obtainedfrom 75% of the peripheral lesions that could not be biopsied trans bronchially.

E. Magnetic resonance imaging has an advantage over CT in mediastinal lesions that aretoo close to the major vessels.

References.1. Harrison's Principles of Internal Medicine - 13th Edition, 2. Davidson's Principlesand Practices of Medicine - 17th Edition.

Question 85 List the systems of and the treatment for middle lobe syndrome.

Middle lobe syndrome. Middle lobe syndrome may result from mediastinal adenitis that chronically obstructs the bronchus to the right middle lobe, resulting in recurrent pneumonia in asetting of partial atelectasis, scarring, and bronchiectasis. The right middle lobe suffers from this disorder more than do other lobes because the primary lesions in the lung and the adenitis are more common on the right, and a collar of lymph nodes surrounds the origin of the right middle lobe at its orifice. The drainage of this lymphoid collar is from the right middle lobe, the right lower lobe, and the lower esophagus.

The list of systems of middle lobe syndrome are:

A. Obstruction of the lumen of the bronchus. 1. Primary carcinoma of the lung. 2. Metastatic carcinoma. 3. Inhaled foreign body. 4. Adenoma of bronchus.

B. Compression of a bronchus by hilar lymphadenopathy. 1. Carcinoma of the lung, 2. Tuberculosis.

3. Sarcoidosis

C. Mucous impaction. 1. Allergic bronchopulmonary aspergillosis. 2. Bronchial asthma.

D. Retained secretions. 1. Postoperative. 2. Respiratory infection, especially in adults with chronic bronchitis. 3. Whooping cough, measles, and laryngotracheobronchitis in children.

Treatment of middle lobe syndrome. 1. Most forms of mediastinal granulomatous adenitis heal spontaneously without complications. 2. When atelectasis occurs with or without pneumonitis, appropriate medications such as corticosteroids, antibiotics, or anti-tuberculous treatment should be given for the causative condition. 3. Physiotherapy is essential for all patients to clear secretions by postural drainage and ancillary methods. 4. When an obstruction is permanent, such as that caused by carcinoma of the bronchus, or a bronchial stricture secondary to a tuberculousprocess, the collapse is permanent. Thus, some degree of bronchiectasis is inevitable.

References. 1. Harrison's Principles of Internal Medicine - 13th Edition,

2. Davidson's Principles and Practices of Medicine - 17th Edition.

Question 86 Discuss the symptomatology of emphysema.

Emphysema. The characteristic symptoms are cough with the production of sputum, wheezing, and breathlessness following many years of a smoker's cough. The patient

may have pursing of lips.
Colds seem to 'go down to the chest,' and frequent infective exacerbations occur, giving purulentsputum. Symptoms can be worsened by factors such as cold, foggy weather, and atmospheric pollution. With advancing disease, the patient will become more breathless with mild activity.

Question 87 Describe the principal postoperative pulmonary complications.

Postoperative pulmonary complications. 1. Acute hemorrhage 2. Deep vein thrombosis 3.Pulmonary embolism 4. Right-sided heart failure due to pulmonary vascular disease.

Question 88 What is the treatment of pulmonary embolism?

Treatment of pulmonary embolism

The basis of treatment is intravenous heparin, a bolus dose of 10,000 units followed by a continuous infusion of 1000 to 2000 units/hr. Start oral anticoagulant after 48 hours, and the heparin is tapered off as the oral anticoagulant becomes effective. The oral anticoagulant is continued for 6 weeks to 6 months, depending on the recurrence of the thrombosis or embolism. Dissolution of the embolism can be done by using fibrinolytic therapy, like streptokinase, 250 000 units by intravenous infusion over 30 minutes, followed by streptokinase 100 000 units intravenous hourly. It can be given into the pulmonary artery. Surgical embolectomy may be used if the hemodynamic conditions are very severe. Inferior vena cavil plication or the insertionof a filter into the inferior vena cava may be used if the anticoagulant or fibrinolytic therapy failsor is contraindicated to prevent the recurrences of pulmonary embolism.

Question 89 List the most common causes of acute mediastinitis.

Most common causes of mediastinitis. 1. Esophageal perforation due to esophagoscopy andinsertion of a Blakemore tube. 2. After median sternotomy for cardiac surgery.

References.

1. Harrison's Principles of Internal Medicine - 13th Edition.

2. Davidson's Principles and Practices of Medicine - 17th Edition,

Question 90 What complicating diseases may occur with a diaphragmatic hernia?

Complicating diseases that occur with a diaphragmatic hernia. 1. Peripheral neuropathies involving the diaphragm. 2. Anterior horn cell disorder, like poliomyelitis 3. Connective tissuedisorders, like systemic lupus erythematous 4. Hypothyroidism and hyperthyroidism may causediaphragmatic weakness. 5. Pulmonary hyperinflation, like emphysema 6. Small stiff lungs, likediffuse pulmonary fibrosis, decrease diaphragmatic efficiency and predispose to fatigue. 7. Severe skeletal deformities, like kyphosis, can cause gross distortions of diaphragmatic muscle configuration.

Question 91 How would you diagnose a pulmonary arteriovenous fistula of hemangioma?

Pulmonary arteriovenous fistula of hemangioma can be diagnosed by:

1. Contrast CT scan
2. Magnetic resonance imaging
3. Digital subtraction pulmonary angiography.

Q. 92 What are the most common complications of acute barbiturate poisoning?

The most common complications of barbiturate poisoning are 1. Central nervous system depressionranging from confusion and lethargy to coma. 2. In severe cases of poisoning, hypotension, hypothermia, pulmonary edema, and cardiac arrest can occur. 3. Bullous skin lesions and pressuresores may occur in severe cases. 4. Hypostatic pneumonia, decubiti, and aspiration may occur in comatose cases. 5. Acute renal failure may occur.

Question 93 Give the principal manifestations of berylliosis (beryllium poisoning).

Beryllium poisoning 1. Ulcerative tracheobronchitis 2. Chemical pneumonitis. 3. Chronicinterstitial pneumonitis. 4. Acute pneumonitis.

Question 94 Define silo-filler's disease.

Silo-filler's disease. It is an acute toxic noncardiogenic pulmonary edema caused by inhalation ofnitrogen dioxide in recently filled silos. It can be treated with corticosteroids to prevent bronchiolitis obliterans. However, sudden death may result if there is chronic exposure to silage gas.

Question 95 What are the most common causes of diseases involving the oral cavity?

Most common diseases involve the oral cavity. 1. Aphthous ulcers 2. Candidiasis. 3. Herpeticstomatitis. 4. Pharyngitis and tonsillitis. 5. Necrotizing ulcerative gingivitis. 6. Leukoplakia and erythroplakia. 7. Oral carcinoma. 8. Glossitis and glossodynia. 9. Peri tonsillitis abscess and cellulitis

Question 96 Discuss the role of teeth in disease.

The role of teeth in disease. 1. Tetracyclines are bound to the calcium deposited in the growingteeth, causing fluorescence, discoloration, enamel dysplasia, deformity, or growth inhibition.
Therefore, tetracycline should not be given to pregnant women or children under 6 years of age. 2. Temporomandibular pain syndrome is a functional disorder of the temporomandibular joint associated with bite abnormalities. This occurs in anxious people who grind their teeth at night, which gives rise to pain and clicking in one or both temporomandibular joints. It can be treated by correction of the bite. 3. Inadequate mastication offood may cause dyspepsia. 4. Gingivitis and apical abscess, and after dental manipulation, can be a source of septicemia and may give rise to bacterial endocarditis in a patient with valvular diseaseof the heart.

Question 97 What are the cause and significance of leukoplakia?

Leukoplakia is a white lesion found in the oral cavity caused by chronic irritations, like dentures and smoking tobacco. It cannot be easily removed by rubbing the mucosal surfaceof the oral cavity. The significance of it is that it may represent dysplasia or early invasive squamous cell carcinoma.

Question 98 Discuss the etiology of xerostomia.

Etiology of xerostomia. 1. Psychogenic, commonly due to anxiety. 2. Pyrexia. 3. Drugs like anticholinergics, antihistamines, and tricyclic antidepressants. 4. Sjogren's syndrome, with dryness of the mouth, vagina, and skin, and keratoconjunctivitis sicca, without rheumatoid arthritis. 5. Diabetic ketoacidosis and dehydration,

Question 99 What condition may cause bleeding gums?

Bleeding gums due to.

1. Gingivitis is caused by the failure to remove bacteria in the form of plaque from the tooth.
2. Bleeding disorders, like deficiency of clotting factors and platelets.
3. Immunocompromised patients and with acute leukemia.
4. Scurvy.

Question 100 Give classification of diseases of the esophagus.

Classification of diseases of the esophagus.

A. Dysphagia 1. The disease of the mouth and tongue, like tonsillitis. 2. Neuromuscular disorders, like Pharyngeal disorders, bulbar palsy, myasthenia gravis, esophageal motility disorders, achalasia,scleroderma, diffuse esophageal spasm, presbyoesophagus, diabetes, Chagas 's disease. 3. Extrinsic pressure, like mediastinal glands, goiter, and enlarged left atrium. 4. Intrinsic lesions, like a.Foreign bodies b. Stricture- Benign- peptic, corrosive.

Malignant- carcinoma. c. Lower esophageal rings- esophageal web, pharyngeal pouch.

B. Heartburn.

C. Painful swallowing

D. Painful dysphagia due to severe reflux esophagitis or infection due to candida or herpessimplex.

E. Esophageal regurgitation.

References. 1. Harrison's Principles of Internal Medicine - 13th Edition. 2. Davidson's Principlesand Practices of Medicine - 17th Edition,

Question 101 What are the etiology, symptomatology, and treatment of esophageal varies?

The etiology of esophageal varies.

1. Secondary to portal hypertension, and the commonest cause of it is cirrhosis.

2. Active alcohol abuse with established alcoholic cirrhosis.

3. Drugs that cause mucosal erosion, like salicylates and other non-steroidal anti-inflammatorydrugs.

Symptomatology of esophageal varices. Patients may present with vomiting of bright red blood or coffee ground material which is accompanied by melena. Sometimes, only melena is presentwithout hematemesis. Severe variceal bleeding may cause hypovolemia with signs of shock.

Many patients may have signs of chronic liver failure, like palmar erythema, spider angiomas,gynecomastia, asterixis, muscle wasting, splenomegaly, ascites, and jaundice.

Treatment of esophageal varices.

A. Acute resuscitation. Variceal bleeding may be a life-threatening emergency. Rapid patient assessment and resuscitation of fluids and blood products are essential. Fresh frozen plasma is to be given to patients with coagulopathy due to cirrhosis. A nasogastric tube is to be inserted into thestomach to reduce nausea and vomiting and to monitor any further bleeding

B. Emergency endoscopy. This should be performed in a patient who has been stabilized hemodynamically to look for other sources of upper gastrointestinal bleeding and to stop any further variceal bleeding, up to 90% of the cases, by sclerotherapy and banding of the varices. The sclerotherapy is done by injecting sclerosing agents, like ethanolamine and tetradecyl sulfate, into the variceal trunks. Then, endoscopic rubber banding of the varices can be performed witha device attached at thc cnd of thc endoscope.

C. Reduction of portal venous pressure. A combination of vasopressin and nitroglycerin can reducethe splanchnic blood flow and decrease the portal venous resistances by lowering the portal pressure by 10 to 40%. Vasopressin can be started at 0.4 units/ min intravenously, and the dosage is tapered after the bleeding is controlled. Nitroglycerin is administered intravenously at a rate of 40 to 400 micrograms/min and titrated to maintain the systolic blood pressure above 90 mm Hg, reducing the vasoconstricting effect of vasopressin which can cause cardiac arrhythmias, myocardial ischemia, mesenteric ischemia, hypertension, bradycardia, and hyponatremia. Octreotide, a synthetic form of somatostatin, may be used in place of vasopressin to reduce portal pressure and stop variceal bleeding. It is given as 50 micrograms intravenously and followed by an infusion of 50 micrograms hourly.

D. Local measures.

1. Balloon tamponade. The Sengstaken-Blakemore tube can control up to 90% of the variceal bleeding but with a rebleeding up to 50%. It has a gastric balloon inflated for 12 to 48 hours to provide the tamponade of the bleeding varices. It is a second-line therapy if thebleeding varices cannot be controlled with endoscopy and pharmacologic measures.

2. Trans jugular intrahepatic portosystemic stent (TIPS). TIPS creates a portosystemic shunt fromthe portal vein to the hepatic vein. TIPS can control bleeding in up to 90% of patients.

E. Emergency portosystemic shunt surgery. Not a preferred choice as hepatic encephalopathyand morbidity and mortality are high for this procedure. It is used for patients if the above measures fail and if the patient has a good liver function.

F. Beta-blockers. Propranolol, 20 to 60 mg twice a day, may be effective in preventing theincidence of rebleeding from esophageal varices and portal hypertensive gastropathy.

Question 102 Differentiate between gastric ulcer and carcinoma. What is the recommended treatment?

	Gastric ulcer	**Gastric Carcinoma**

Incidence	About 20% of adult population	About 15% of all cancer deaths
Sites	Mostly in the lesser curvatureof the stomach	50% from the pyloric region and 25% from the lesser curvature.
Etiology and risk factors	NSAIDs, Chronic H. pylori infection, Acid hypersecretory states, like Zollinger-Ellison syndrome	Chronic H. pylori gastritis, Chronic atrophic gastritis with intestinal metaplasia, Pernicious anemia, Partial gastric resection >15 yearsago
Clinical features	Clinical Epigastric pain with nausea and vomiting, Nocturnal pain that awakens the patient. Fecal occult blood positive	Vomiting, weight loss, dyspepsia, anorexia. It may be agastric mass felt. Melena or hematemesis, Guaiac-positive stools
Blood test	Anemia if bleeding ulcer.	Iron deficiency anemia due to chronic blood loss
Endoscopy	Done with biopsy for H. pylori gastritis.	Done with cytologic brushing and biopsy

<u>Treatment for gastric ulcer.</u>

Treatment is given to ensure ulcer healing and to check with a follow-up endoscopy and biopsy at 6 weeks. Failure to heal should raise the question of malignancy. 1. **Gastric ulcer** attributed to Helicobacter pylori infection. a. Ranitidine 150 mg twice daily for 6 to 8 weeks withthe "triple regimen" for 2 weeks. The triple regimen is bismuth 600 mg four times a day, metronidazole 250 mg four times a day, and tetracycline 500 mg four times a day. Or b. Omeprazole 20-40 mg twice daily for 4 to 6 weeks with amoxicillin 500 mg four times daily orclarithromycin 500 mg three times daily for two weeks. 2.

Gastric ulcer not attributed to Helicobacter pylori infection and may be due to NSAIDS and Zollinger-Ellison syndrome. a. Cimetidine 800 mg nocte or 400 mg twice daily, Ranitidine or nizatidine 300 mg noctre or 150 mg twice daily, or Famotidine 40 mg nocte or 20 mg twice daily for 6 to 8 weeks. b. Omeprazole 40 mg daily for 6 to 8 weeks. And add sucralfate 1 gram four times daily for 6 to 8 weeks. 3. Surgery is rarely performed due to the effective medication treatment. Two types of surgery are partial gastrectomy and vagotomy.

Treatment for gastric carcinoma.

Surgery is the only available therapy with curative potential. Patients with localized carcinoma without distant metastasis and adjacent organ spread who have undergone complete resection may have a 20 to 30 % 5-year survival rate. For distal tumors, curative resection consists of subtotal gastrectomy and regional lymphadenectomy. For proximal tumors, total gastrectomy withsplenectomy is done, and Palliative resection is done for advanced gastric carcinoma, which isassociated with longer survival and better quality of life.

Question 103 Outline the management of

uncomplicated peptic ulcer.

Management of uncomplicated peptic ulcer.

Treatment is given to ensure ulcer healing and to check with a follow-up of endoscopy andbiopsy at 6 weeks.

1. Helicobacter pylori associated with peptic ulcer. a. Ranitidine 150 mg twice daily for 6 to 8 weeks with the triple regimen for 2 weeks. The triple regimen is bismuth 600 mg four times a day, metronidazole 250 mg four times a day, and tetracycline 500 mg four times a day. Or b. Omeprazole 20-40 mg twice daily for 4 to 6 weeks with amoxicillin 500 mg four times daily or clarithromycin 500 mg three times daily for two weeks.

2. Peptic ulcer is not due to H. pylori and may be due to NSAIDs and Zollinger-Ellison syndrome.
a. Cimetidine 800 mg noctre or 400 mg twice daily, Ranitidine or nizatidine 300 mg noctre or150 mg twice daily, or Famotidine 40 mg noctre or 20 mg twice daily for 6 to 8 weeks. b. Omeprazole 40 mg daily for 6 to 8 weeks. And add sucralfate 1 gram four times daily for 6 to 8 weeks.

3. Smoking should be stopped as smokers have a high incidence of peptic ulcer. Dietary changesare not necessary.

4. NSAIDs should be stopped in patients with peptic ulcer. However, this may not be possible in patientswho are dependent on NSAIDs for severe arthritis. Therefore, NSAIDs may be continued with ranitidine or misoprostol together.

Question 104 What measures are employed to

prevent ulcer recurrences?

Measures to prevent ulcer recurrences.

1. Eradication of Helicobacter pylori prevents 90% of ulcer recurrences. Therefore, treat allpatients with a "triple regimen" or omeprazole and an antibiotic, like amoxicillin or clarithromycin for 2 weeks to eradicate H. Pylori.

2. To stop NSAIDs and to treat NSAIDs-induced ulcer with Misoprostol 100-200 microgramsfour times daily or Ranitidine 150 mg twice daily.

3. Chronic daily maintenance may be given to patients with a. Recurrent H. pylori-negative ulcers due to NSAIDs. b. Recurrent ulcers in which H. pylori cannot be successfullytreated. c. Patients with a previous history of ulcer bleeding. Ranitidine 150 mg, cimetidine 400 mg, famotidine 20 mg noctre.

References.

1. Harrison's Principles of Internal Medicine - 13th Edition.
2. Davidson's Principles and Practices of Medicine - 17th Edition.

Question 105 Give symptoms and differential diagnosis of regional enteritis (terminal ileitis Crohn's disease).

Symptoms of regional enteritis.

Major symptoms are diarrhea, abdominal pain, and weight loss. The other constitutional symptoms of malaise, lethargy, anorexia, nausea, vomiting, and low-grade fever may be present. The disease can be insidious or acute. The abdominal pain may be colicky and localized to the lower right quadrant, but sometimes it may be only minimal discomfort. Ifthere is associated intestinal obstruction, there may be cramping abdominal pains, postprandial bloating, and loud borborygmi. Diarrhea is present in 80% of all cases, often intermittent in nature, and it may be associated with blood. Some patients, about 15%, may only present with anorexia, weight loss, and general ill health without the absence of other gastrointestinal symptoms. There may be features of perianal abscess and fistula and anal fissures.

Differential diagnosis of regional enteritis. 1. Ulcerative colitis. 2. Appendicitis. 3. Other causesof ileitis, like infection with Yersinia enterocolitica enteritis. 4. Irritable bowel syndrome. 5.
Intestinal lymphoma. 6. AIDS patients with fever and diarrhea. 7. Segmental colitis due to tuberculosis, Entamoeba histolytica, Chlamydia, or ischemic colitis. 8. Diverticulitis with abscessformation.

Question 106 Define malabsorption syndrome.

Malabsorption syndrome.

Malabsorption syndrome is associated with a large variety of small intestinal mucosal diseaseprocesses, which results in malabsorption of nutrients by the gastrointestinal tract, such as pancreatic insufficiency, bile salt insufficiency, and postsurgical abnormalities.

Question 107 Discuss the etiology, clinical manifestations, and treatment of pseudomembranousenterocolitis and staphylococcal enteritis.

Pseudomembranous enterocolitis.

Etiology. It is caused by the A and B toxins produced by Clostridium difficile. It is usually occurring a few days after antibiotics therapy or, sometimes a month after discontinuing the antibiotics. The usual antibiotics causing this condition are clindamycin, ampicillin, tetracycline,and cephalosporins.

Clinical manifestations. Fever, diarrhea, and abdominal cramps. The sigmoidoscopic examination may show an erythematous, ulcerated mucosa covered with a membrane-like material.

Treatment. Stop all suspected antibiotics may stop diarrhea. Vancomycin 125 mg orally fourtimes daily for 10 days or metronidazole are often used. Patients should be isolated to prevent the spread to other patients.

Staphylococcal enteritis.

Etiology. It is caused by staphylococcus aureus that disrupts the normal absorption and secretoryprocess in the small intestine.

Clinical manifestations.

Watery, nonblood diarrhea associated with periumbilical cramps, bloating, nausea, and vomiting.Diarrhea may be severe and result in dehydration with hypokalemia and metabolic acidosis due to loss of HCO3- in the stool.

Treatment.

1. Take adequate oral fluids containing carbohydrates and electrolytes. Rest the bowel byavoiding high-fiber foods, fats, milk products, caffeine, and alcohol.
2. Rehydration with oral electrolyte solutions. Intravenous fluids, lactated Ringer's solution, for the patient with severe dehydration and unable to tolerate orally.
3. Antidiarrhea agents, like loperamide 4 mg stat dose,

followed by 2 mg thereafter, with amaximum of 16 mg/24 hours.

4. Antibiotic treatment should not be warranted.

Question 108 List the common disturbance of the colon.

The common disturbance of the colon. 1. Diverticular disease. 2. Antibiotic-associated diarrhea.
3. Inflammatory bowel disease- Ulcerative colitis and Crohn's disease 4. Pseudomembranous colitis. 5. Colonic benign polyps and colonic carcinoma. 6. Familial adenomatous polyposis 7. Irritable bowel syndrome. 8. Constipation, 9. Fecal impaction. 10. Laxative abuse syndrome

Question 109 Differentiate between cerebral vomiting and gastric vomiting.

Cerebral vomiting.

Disorder of the central nervous system (CNS) or certain sights, smells, or emotional experiencesmay induce vomiting like:

1. Increased intracranial pressure due to CNS tumors, subdural or subarachnoid hemorrhage.
2. Infections like meningitis and encephalitis.
3. Vestibular disorders like Meniere's syndrome, labyrinthitis, and motion sickness.
4. Psychogenic, like bulimia, psychiatric disorders, and anticipatory vomiting.

Gastric vomiting

Stimulation of the afferent vagal fibers and splanchnic fibers from the gastrointestinal viscera bygastrointestinal distension or infections.

1. Gastric mechanical obstruction, like peptic ulcer disease and malignancy.
2. Gastric dysmotility, like gastroparesis due to diabetes, medications, post viral and post vagotomy.
3. Infections, like viral gastroenteritis, food poisoning by toxins, hepatitis A or B, and acutesystemic infections.
4. Gastric irritants, like alcohol, oral antibiotics, and NSAIDs.

Question 110 What is the value of peritoneoscopy?

The value of peritoneoscopy. Peritoneoscopy can be used under general and local anesthesia.It provides the visualization of the abdominal cavity and the pelvic cavity via a sub-umbilical incision. It can be used for diagnosis, biopsies, treatment, and tubal ligation for sterilization. It also provides a good view of the liver, gallbladder, spleen, the prominent blood vessels of portalhypertension, and any evidence of peritoneal diseases.

Question 111 Differentiate intestinal colic, uterine colic, and renal colic.

Intestinal colic	**Uterine colic**	**Renal colic**
Acute paroxysmal abdominalpain arising from the colon.	Severe colic arises in the uterusduring the menstrual period.	Pain due to thrombosis of the renal artery or vein, dissection of the renal artery, renal infarction, intrarenal mass lesion, or passage of a stone within the collecting system

Question 112 What is Virchow's node or signal node?

Virchow's node is a palpable lymph node sometimes found in the supraclavicular fossa seen inthe stomach carcinoma.

Question 113 Discuss the management of chronic ulcerative colitis.

Management of chronic ulcerative colitis.

1. Oral corticosteroids. Oral prednisolone 40 to 60 mg daily can be given for 3 to 6 weeks, depending on the response. Corticosteroids can induce remission in the majority of patients, and the dose is reduced at weekly intervals over 4 weeks as improvement occurs. Corticosteroidsgive rise to a sense of well-being and improve appetite, enabling the problem of persuading the patient to eat enough food. However, long-term use is associated with serious, potentially irreversible side-effects and is to be avoided.

2. Azathioprine. Azathioprine, 2.5 mg/kg daily, may be helpful in patients with chronic diseasefor whom the surgery is inappropriate. It has advantage in reducing the dose of corticosteroids in patients with troublesome side effects of corticosteroids. However, it has its side-effects like bone marrow suppression with pancytopenia.

3. Surgery. Surgery is indicated in chronic disease, where the disease leaves a permanently damaged bowel with stricture formation. A chronic disease of more than 10 years may risk of carcinoma. Therefore, a serious consideration for proctocolectomy, especially if a precancerous lesion is detected on routine colonoscopy. A

full explanation of the ileostomy andits management with the actual appliance should be demonstrated to the patient. If the rectum is not grossly involved, then it may be preserved and ileorectal anastomosis performed.

4. Ulcerative colitis is a lifelong illness that has many social and emotional impacts on patients. Patients should be encouraged to join the Crohn's and Colitis Foundation of America foremotional and social support from others with a similar illness.

References.

1. Harrison's Principles of Internal Medicine - 13th Edition,
2. Davidson's Principles and Practices of Medicine - 17th Edition

Question 114 Differentiate diverticulitis and carcinoma of the sigmoid.

Diverticulitis

Diverticulitis is the inflammation of the diverticula. It is mostly found in the sigmoid colon but can be presented in the whole colon. Diverticulitis occurs when the feces obstruct the neck of thediverticulum, causing stagnation and allowing bacteria to multiply and produce inflammation.
This can lead to bowel perforation (peri diverticulitis), abscess formation, fistulas into adjacentorgans, or even generalized peritonitis.

Clinical features.

Severe pain in the left iliac fossa accompanied by fever and constipation. There will be tenderness, guarding, and rigidity on the left side of the abdomen. Complication. 1. Abscess formation 2. Perforation with generalized peritonitis. 3. Fistula formation into the bladder or the vagina. 4. Intestinal obstruction. Treatment. Bowel rest, intravenous fluids and antibiotics, cephalosporin, and metronidazole. Surgery consists of DE functioning colostomy for intestinal obstruction and fistulae.

Carcinoma of sigmoid.

It has a genetic inheritance in developing sigmoid carcinoma. There is a two to three increased lifetime risk of developing sigmoid carcinoma with one first-degree affected family member.This tumor is a polypoid mass with ulceration and spreads by direct infiltration through the bowel wall and invades the lymphatics and the blood vessels with early spread to the liver.

Clinical features

Alteration of bowel habits with or without abdominal pain. The stool is usually mixed withblood. There may be intestinal obstruction. A mass may be felt on examination,

Treatment

Surgical resection and end-to-end anastomosis. The 5-year survival rate is 30%.Chemotherapy may be used if there is metastasis and surgery is inappropriate.

Question 115 How would you make a diagnosis of tuberculous peritonitis?

Diagnosis of tuberculous peritonitis.

A. Examination of the peritoneal fluid for 1. Increase of lymphocytes. 2. Tubercle bacilli on staining. 3. Culture of the fluid. B. Ultrasound of the abdomen may show a mesenteric thickening and enlarged lymph nodes. C. Laparoscopic examination of the abdomen may showthat the peritoneum is studded with tubercles sent for biopsy and culture.

Question 116 Name five extra-abdominal diseases which may stimulate an acute surgical abdomen.

The five extra-abdominal diseases. 1. Myocardial infarction as in referred pain. 2. Pneumonia asin referred pain, 3. Porphyria. 4. Lead poisoning. 5. Diabetes mellitus with ketoacidosis.

Question 117 Differentiate between diabetic acidosis and appendicitis.

Diabetic acidosis.

It is a state of uncontrolled catabolism associated with insulin deficiency. This a metabolic emergency in which hyperglycemia is associated with metabolic acidosis due to raised ketonelevels.

Clinical features.

The patient will present with prostration, hyperventilating (Kussmaul respiration), nausea, vomiting, and abdominal pain, which may add to the confusion of an acute abdomen.

Diagnosis.

Demonstration of hyperglycemia with

ketonemia or heavy ketonuria and acidosis.

Treatment.

1. Replacement of fluids, electrolytes, and insulin.
2. Monitoring the blood glucose closely.
3. Replacement of energy losses.

Complications
1. Hypotension with renal failure.
2. Cerebral edema and coma.
3. Stasis pneumonia and deep vein thrombosis.

Appendicitis. Acute appendicitis is mostly due to the obstruction of the lumen of the appendixwith a fecolith, and sometimes only a generalized inflammation.

Clinical features. Abdominal pain starts in the center of the abdomen and is later localized to the right iliac fossa. There may be nausea, vomiting, and occasional diarrhea. There may be guardingdue to localized peritonitis.

Diagnosis. Demonstration of an increased white cell count and use of ultrasound to show theinflamed appendix or an appendix mass. The surgically excised appendix should be sent for histology.

Treatment. Surgery-appendicectomy.

Complications. Perforation of the inflamed appendix with gangrene formation, leading to alocalized abscess or generalized peritonitis.

References.

1. Harrison's Principles of Internal Medicine - 13th Edition. 2
2. Davidson's Principles and Practices of Medicine - 17th Edition.

Question 118 Give the etiology and management of constipation,

Etiology of constipation. 1. Simple constipation due to low fiber intake. 2. Drugs like opiates, codeine, iron, antidepressants, and aluminum antacids. 3. Intestinal obstruction. 4. Colonic disease, like carcinoma. 5. Painful anal conditions. 6. Hypothyroidism and hypercalcemia. 7. Depressionand immobility. 8. Hirschsprung's disease.

Management of constipation. Take a high-fiber diet. Bulking agents, like methylcellulose and branshould be tried first. Glycerol suppositories and enemas may be used. Stimulant laxatives are for short-term use only as they may cause cramps and atonic non-functioning colon in long-term use. Osmotic laxatives, like magnesium sulfate and lactulose, can be used for severe constipation.
Treat the underlying cause of constipation.

Question 119 What is the significance of a "rectal shelf"?

Significance of a "rectal shelf." "Rectal shelf" is a sign of metastatic spread of carcinoma. Thus, this significant sign should prompt the clinician to investigate immediately for a primarysource of **carcinoma.**

Question 120 Give classification of diseases of the liver.

Classification of diseases of the liver. The classification can be divided into acute and chronicliver diseases.

Acute liver diseases.

1. Viral infections (Hepatitis A, B, C, D, E, Cytomegalovirus, Epstein-Barr virus, Herpes simplex virus, Yellow fever virus.)

2. Post-viral infection (Reye ‘s syndrome)

3. Non-viral infections (Leptospira icterohemorrhagiae, Coxiella burneti, Toxoplasma gonadii)

4. Drugs like halothane and acetaminophen

5. Poisons. a. Amanita phalloides mushroom. b. Carbon tetrachloride.

6. Metabolic a. Wilson's disease. b. Fatty change in pregnancy

7. Ischemic a. Shock b. Severe cardiac failure or tamponade. c. Budd-Chiari syndrome

Chronic liver diseases

1. Infections Hepatitis B, C, D
2. Toxins (Alcohol and Drugs like methyldopa, isoniazid)
3. Biliary obstruction (Primary biliary cirrhosis, Primary sclerosing cholangitis, Secondarybiliary cirrhosis due to stone, stricture, neoplasm)
4. Metabolic diseases. (Hemochromatosis, Wilson's disease, Alpha-antitrypsin deficiency)
5. Fibrocystic disease
6. Nutritional (Intestinal bypass surgery)
7. Hepatic congestion (Budd-Chiari syndrome, Veno-occlusive disease, Cardiac failure)

Question 121 Define "Charcot's intermittent hepatic fever."

Charcot's intermittent hepatic fever. It is part of a combination of a triad which consists of pain,fever, and jaundice of cholangitis.

Question 122 Give the etiology and treatment of biliary dyskinesia.

Etiology of biliary dyskinesia.

1. Spasm of the sphincter of Oddi
2. Denervation sensitivity resulting in hypertonicity of the

gallbladder,
3. Abnormalities of the sequencing or frequency rates of sphincter contraction waves.

Treatment.

1. Medical- nitrites or anticholinergics to relax the sphincter of Oddi.
2. Surgical sphincteroplasty or endoscopic sphincterotomy for patients who do not respond to themedical treatment.

Question 123 What is "syringe" jaundice?

"Syringe" jaundice. It is the way Hepatitis B and C viruses spread by means of the intravenous route,such as contaminated needles used by drug addicts, tattooists, or acupuncturists and resulting in acute hepatitis with jaundice.

Question 124 Give the clinical significance of carotenemia.

Clinical significance of carotenemia. An excess intake of beta-carotenes from colored vegetablesmay result in benign staining of the skin, a yellowish-orange color on the palms, and soles, while the sclera remains white, which distinguishes it from jaundice.

Question 125 Of what value is Courvoisier "law"?

Courvoisier "law." A jaundiced patient with a palpable, sometimes visible dilated gallbladdershould lead the clinician to suspect and investigate for carcinoma of the head of the pancreas.

References. 1. Harrison's Principles of Internal Medicine - 13th Edition. 2. Davidson's Principlesand Practices of

Medicine - 17th Edition.

Q. 126 Differentiate between epidemic infectious (virus A) jaundice and homologous serum jaundice (virus B).

	Epidemic infectious (virus A)	Homologous serum jaundice (virus B)
Virus	Picornavirus Rna Virus	Hepadnavirus DNA virus
Spread	Feco-oral saliva	Blood, saliva, vertical and sexual
Incubation	Short 2-3 weeks	Long 1-5 months
Age	Young	Any
Carrier state	No	Yes
Chronic liver disease	No	Yes
Liver carcinoma	No	Yes
Mortality (acute)	<0.5%	<1%
Immunization (Active)	Vaccine	Vaccine
Immunization (Passive)	Normal immunoglobulin	Hepatitis B immunoglobulin (HBIG) vaccine

<u>References.</u>

1. Harrison's Principles of Internal Medicine - 13th Edition,
2. Davidson's Principles and Practices of Medicine - 17th Edition.

Question 127 Outline the management of cirrhosis of the liver.

<u>Management of cirrhosis of the liver.</u> There is no treatment to reverse cirrhosis and to ensure thatthere is no further progression occurs. However, medical treatment can

improve general health and alleviate symptoms. The main aim is to:

A. Detect treatable causes, such as alcohol abuse, drug ingestion, hemochromatosis, and Wilson'sdisease. Abstinence from alcohol is very important.

B. To prevent and correct malnutrition. In the absence of encephalopathy or ascites, a high-energy(3000 kcal/d), protein-rich (80 100 g/d) diet should be advised. If there is no cholestasis, fat intake need not be restricted. If there is fluid retention, then the salt restriction is necessary.

C. To manage chronic cholestasis. Cholestyramine to relieve pruritus. Steatorrhea can be reducedby limiting fat intake. Malabsorption of fat-soluble vitamins and calcium is treated with a monthly injection of vitamin K, oral vitamin D, and oral calcium supplement.

D. To treat certain complications. 1. Ascites and edema due: a. Sodium retention - Restriction ofdietary sodium intake to 400-800 mg/d. Spironolactone should be used if there is no respond to salt restriction alone. b. Hypoproteinemia - Restoration of plasma protein depends on improving liver function. Therefore, intravenous albumin is of little value. c. Portal hypertension - Large volume paracentesis (4-6 L) may be needed if respiratory is compromised and in massive ascites. Concomitantly, to give intravenous albumin, 8-10 g/L of ascites fluid was removed to protect the intravascular volume. Trans jugular intrahepatic portosystemic shunts (TIPS) for severe ascites.

2. Hepatic encephalopathy: The dietary protein should be withheld during the acute phase. Lactulose 30 mL three to four times daily and neomycin sulfate, 0,5-1 g

orally every 6 or 12hours for 5-7 days to decrease the amount of ammonia produced to decrease neurotoxicity. Avoid narcotics, tranquilizers, and sedatives, which are metabolized by the liver.

3. Anemia: Iron tablets for iron deficiency anemia and folic acid supplement in macrocyticanemia due to alcoholism.

4. Hemorrhagic tendency: Can be treated by vitamin K preparation, transfusion of packed redblood cells, and fresh-frozen plasma.

5. Hemorrhage from esophageal varices: Hemorrhage may be arrested by injection of sclerotherapy and band ligation endoscopically, balloon tamponade, or intravenous vasopressinwith nitroglycerin,

6. Spontaneous bacterial peritonitis: Initiate antibiotics, cefotaxime 2 g intravenously every 8hours for 5-10 days.

E. Liver transplantation is done in selected cases of irreversible, progressive, chronic liver disease, fulminant hepatic failure, and certain metabolic diseases in which the metabolic defect isin the liver. It should also be considered in patients with worsening functional status, rising bilirubin, decreasing albumin, coagulopathy, refractory ascites, recurrent variceal bleeding, or worsening encephalopathy.

Question 128 Describe methods of lowering blood ammonia in hepatic coma.

Methods of lowering blood ammonia in hepatic coma.

1. In the acute phase of hepatic coma, dietary protein should be stopped, thus

decreasing the ammonia by-product in the blood.

2. Lactulose is digested by the bacteria in the colon to short-chain fatty acids, resulting in acidification of the colonic content. This acidification forms ammonium which is not absorbable and thus is not toxic. Lactulose also leads to the change of ammonia-forming organisms resulting in less ammonia formed neurotoxic. Lactulose 30 mL is giventhree to four times daily, and the dose is titrated so that patient has only two to three soft stools per day.

3. Neomycin sulfate 0.5 g orally every 6 to 12 hours for 5 to 7 days which can control the ammonia-producing intestinal flora.

4. Upper gastrointestinal bleeding should be controlled, and blood should be purged from the gastrointestinal tract. The nasogastric tube is used or magnesium citrate orally 120 mL every3-4 hours until the stool is free from gross blood.

Question 129 What is the Cruveilhier-Baumgarten syndrome.

Cruzeilhier-Baumgarten Syndrome. It is the venous hum heard on auscultation of the large umbilical collateral vessel, with a large blood flow, which is a part of the dilated collateral vessels on the anterior wall of the abdomen resulting from portal hypertension.

Question 130 What is the treatment for silent gallstones?

Silent or asymptomatic gallstones are usually not

treated because most will nevergive symptoms. Therefore, there is no need for a prophylactic cholecystectomy in an asymptomatic person.

Question 131 What is the relative frequency of carcinoma in ascending, transverse,descending, and sigmoid portions of the colon and in the rectum?

Frequency of carcinoma.
1. Ascending colon - 19%
2. Transverse colon - 18%
3. Descending colon - 8%
4. Sigmoid portion of the colon - 29%
5. Rectum - 26%

Question 132 What is the value of a liver biopsy? How may it be obtained?

Value of liver biopsy. A liver biopsy is a valuable histological examination of the liver in thedifferential diagnosis of diffuse or localized parenchymal disease. The indications for liver biopsy are A. Liver disease 1. Unexplained hepatomegaly 2. Persistently abnormal liver biochemistry 3. Cirrhosis 4. Drug-related liver disease 5. Tumors - primary or secondary 6.Systemic disease. B. Screening relatives of patients with certain diseases, such as hemochromatosis C. Pyrexia of unknown origin.

A liver biopsy is performed under ultrasound or CT control when a localized lesion in the liver needs to be biopsied. Laparoscopy with guided liver biopsy is performed through a small incision in the abdominal wall under local anesthesia.

Question 133 Give the differential diagnosis of acute cholecystitis.

Differential diagnosis of acute cholecystitis.
1. Perforated peptic ulcer.
2. Retrocecal appendicitis.
3. Acute appendicitis.
4. Right basal pneumonia,
5. Myocardial infarction.

Question 134 What is mucoviscidosis?

Mucoviscidosis is cystic fibrosis of the pancreas.

Question 135 Differentiate abscess of the liver and cancer of the liver.

Abscess of the liver. The liver abscess can be single or multiple.

Causes. 1. Biliary sepsis. 2. Bacteremia and direct extension from, such as a perinephricabscess. 3. Trauma and portal pyemia from intra-abdominal sepsis.

Pathogens. 1. E. coli - commonest 2. Others - Streptococcus faecalis, Proteus vulgaris, Staphylococcal aureus, Bacteroides and Streptococcus milleri.

Clinical features. It may present as malaise for a few days or_may present more acutely withfever, rigors, anorexia, vomiting, weight loss, and abdominal pain. The patient may be jaundiced with a tender enlarged liver.

Investigations. Ultrasound is very useful in detecting fluid-filled lesions in the liver. CT scanningis used for further localization. Blood cultures are only positive in 30% of cases.

Treatment. Antibiotics cover Gram-positive, Gram-negative, and anaerobic organisms u1the causative organism is identified. Aspiration of the abscess under ultrasound guidance.

Caner of the Liver Causes

1. Carriers of Hepatitis B and C viruses.
2. Other forms of cirrhosis, such as alcoholic cirrhosis and hemochromatosis.
3. Others - androgenic steroids, aflatoxin.

Clinical features Can present with weight loss, anorexia, fever, ache in the right hypochondrium, and ascites. An enlarged, irregular, tender liver may be felt.

Investigations. Liver biopsy under ultrasound guidance for diagnosis. Serum alpha-fetoprotein is raised. Ultrasound may show filling defects in 90% of cases.

Treatment. Surgical resection is occasionally possible. Chemotherapy and radiotherapy arenot helpful. The prognosis is very poor, and survival is less than 6 months.

References

1. Harrison's Principles of Internal Medicine - 13th Edition,
2. Davidson's Principles and Practices of Medicine - 17th Edition.

Question 136 Define and give treatment for "dumping syndrome"?

Dumping syndrome. It is due to the "dumping" of food into the jejunum, which is followed by a rapiddilution of the high osmotic load, and this is seen in patients following gastrectomy or gastroenterostomy. The patient may present with nausea, vomiting, sweating, faintness, palpitations, and abdominal distension. Many patients learn to cope with it. Treatmentwould involve reassurance and symptomatic therapy, and further surgery is rarely needed.

Question 137 What are the causes of deficiency diseases?

<u>Causes of deficiency diseases</u>. 1. Sepsis 2. Trauma. 3. Surgery - ileal resection. 4. Gastrointestinal diseases - small bowel diseases, ileal diseases, liver, and biliary tract disease 5. Psychological - anorexia nervosa, depression. 6. Dementia 7. Malignancy 8. Metabolic disease -renal failure 9. Very ill patient DO. Decreased intake - alcohol dependency, vegans, elderly withpoor diet. 11. Drugs - oral antibiotics and drug antagonists.

Question 138 Discuss the development of undernutrition.

<u>The development of undernutrition.</u> In developed countries, the leading cause of undernutrition is due to poor intake secondary to anorexia associated with the underlying condition, such as increased catabolism in the septic patient, cachectic cancer patients, and malabsorption in patients with gastrointestinal diseases. In developing countries, undernutrition is due to long-term near-total starvation in adults and children. The protein- energy undernutrition in children manifests in two ways, such as kwashiorkor which occurs ina young child displaced from breast feeding by a new baby and fed with a diet with low protein content, and marasmus is the childhood form of starvation. Both conditions have a deficiency in total calorie intake and other nutrients.

Question 139 List the common causes and clinical manifestations of a deficiency in sodium.

<u>The common cause of a deficiency of sodium</u>

1. Gastrointestinal - "Vomiting, diarrhea, ileostomy losses

2. Renal – Diuretic use Impaired tubular sodium conservation
    - Reflux nephropathy
    - Papillary necrosis - analgesic nephropathy, diabetes, sickle cell disease

3.Burns

4. Hemorrhage

Clinical manifestations of deficiency of sodium

A deficiency of sodium would also affect the loss of water, thus causing shrinkage of the interstitial space and of the blood volume, and thus profound effects on organ functions.

1. Symptoms - Thirst, muscle cramps, nausea, vomiting, and postural dizziness. Severe circulating volume depletion causes hypotension and impairs cerebral perfusion, causingconfusion and coma
2. Signs - Loss of skin elasticity, postural hypotension, peripheral vasoconstriction with cold skin and collapsed peripheral veins, and arterial hypotension_

Question 140 Give the clinical and electrocardiographic manifestations of hypopotassemia.

Manifestation of hypopotassemia

In patients with mild to moderate hypopotassemia, three may be muscular 'weakness, fatigue,muscle cramps, and constipation or ileus_ Severe hypopotassemia may result in flaccid paralysis, hyporeflexia, tetany, and rhabdomyolysis.

Electrocardiographic of hypopotassemia

Decreased amplitude and broadening of the T waves, prominent 1U waves, depressed ST segments_ In severe hypopotassemia „ atrioventricular block and cardiac arrest may occur.

Question 141 In what conditions may a deficiency in vitamin A occur?

Conditions in which deficiency of vitamin A. may occur. 1. Chronic illness with fat malabsorption 2 Severe protein-energy malnutrition. 3. Poor intake of dark green leafy vegetables and carotene-rich fruits in pregnant women and preschool children in developing countries.

Question 142 Give the clinical signs of vitamin B_1 deficiency

Clinical signs of vitamin B_1 deficiency

A. Dry Beriberi
   Patient present with heaviness and stiffness of the legs, followed by weakness, numbness, and pins and needles due to polyneuropathy. The ankle reflexes are lost, adcerebral involvement produces the picture of Wernicke- Korsakoff syndrome.
B. Wet Beriberi
   Patients start to present with ankle edema, which extends to the whole body, with ascites and pleural effusions. The heart muscles may be affected, producing heart failure.
C. Infantile Beriberi
   The infant becomes anorexic and develops

edema and some aphonia. Tachycardia and tachypnea develop, and the condition can become fatal if treatment is given.

Question 143 Outline the treatment of pellagra

Treatment of pellagra Nicotinamide 100 mg every 6 hours orally and a maintenance dose of 50mg daily. The response to the treatment is rapid, with the erythema of the skin diminishing, diarrhea ceasing, and improvement of the patient's behavior and mental altitude. There would beother associated nutritional deficiencies. Therefore, nicotinamide should be supplemented with a nutritious diet high in protein, vitamin B complex, iron, folic acid, and vitamin B12. Alcohol should be avoided.

Question 144 Of what value is pyridoxine in INH toxicity?

The INH toxicity would result in peripheral neuropathy due to secondary pyridoxine(vitamin B_6) deficiency. Therefore, pyridoxine is always given together with INH to prevent peripheral neuropathy

Question 145 Outline the prophylaxis of rickets

Prophylaxis of rickets

1. Education to ensure a balanced diet
2. Exposure to sunlight
3. Taking vitamin D supplements, 10 micrograms (400 i.u) daily

Question 146 Give a practical classification of diseases of the heart.

Classification of diseases of the heart.

A. Congenital heart diseases. 1. Persistent ductus

arteriosus 2. Coarctation of aorta 3. Atrial septal defect 4. Ventricular septal defect 5. Tetralogy of Fallot 6. Others - Transposition of the great arteries, total anomalous pulmonary venous drainage, and tricuspid atresia.

B. Diseases of the heart valves. 1. Rheumatic heart disease 2. Mitral valve disease 3. Aorticvalve disease 4. Tricuspid valve disease 5. Pulmonary valve disease 6. Infective endocarditis.
C. Coronary heart disease and heart
D. Disorders of heart rate rhythm and conduction 1. Atrial tachyarrhythmias 2. Junctional tachyarrhythmias 3. Ventricular tachyarrhythmias 4. Sinoatrial disease 5. Atrioventricularand bundle branch block.
E. Diseases of the myocardium 1. Cardiomyopathy - Dilated, Restrictive, and Hypertrophic.
   2. Cardiac tumors - Atrial myxoma 3. Specific diseases of the heart muscle. a. infections-
   - Viral - e.g., HIV, coxsackie A and B
   Bacterial - e.g. Diphtheria Protozoan-e.g. Trypanosomiasis b. Endocrine and metabolic disorders - e.g., Diabetes, hypo- and hyperthyroidism, acromegaly, carcinoid syndrome, inherited storage diseases. c. Connective tissue diseases-e.g., Scleroderma, SLE, and polyarteritis nodosa. d. Infiltrative disorders - e.g., Hemochromatosis, hemosiderosis, sarcoidosis, amyloidosis. e. Endomyocardial fibrosis and eosinophilic heart disease. f. Toxins - e.g., drugs, alcohol irradiation. g Neuromuscular disorders - e.g., Dystrophia myotonia, Friedreich's ataxia.
F. Diseases of the pericardium. 1. Acute pericarditis 2. Pericardial effusion 3. Tuberculouspericarditis 4. Chronic constrictive pericarditis

Question 147 Give the area of normal heart dullness. What conditions increase the area of

heartdullness?

<u>Area of normal heart dullness.</u> 1. Right border- just immediately to the right lateral border of the stern chondral junction. 2. Base - upper border of the manubrium of the sternum. 3. Apical - in the fifth left intercostal space in the midclavicular line or usually within 10 cm of the midsternalline.

<u>Conditions that increase the area of heart dullness</u> 1. Left ventricular enlargement. 2. Cardiomyopathy 3. Pericardial effusion or tamponade 4. Ventricular aneurysm S. Dilated and elongated arteriosclerotic aorta. 6. Aorta aneurysm, including dissecting aneurysm or syphiliticaneurysm.

Question 148 What are hemic murmurs as applied to the heart, and what is their cause?

Hemic murmurs and their cause. Anemia, hyperthyroidism, and pregnancy may produce a hemic murmur, a short systolic ejection murmur best heard at the left sternal edge. These murmurs could be emanated from the pulmonary or aortic valve.

Question 149 State where topographically mitral and tricuspid murmurs are most distinctlyheard.

Mitral murmur is most distinctly heard in the apex of the heart in the left fifth intercostal space in the midclavicular line. Tricuspid murmur is most distinctly heard over theleft sternal edge.

Question 150 List the etiological factors in the chronic vascular cardia and give an example of each.

Etiologic factors in chronic valvular cardia. 1. Congenital - e.g., Tetralogy of Fallot's 2. Chronic rheumatic carditis - progression fibrosis affecting the heart valves. 3. Infective endocarditis - e.g.,caustic pathogens - Streptococci 4. Syphilitic aortitis 5. Valve ring dilatation - e.g., dilated cardiomyopathy 6. Senile degeneration

Question 151 Give the physical signs of the most usual valvular lesion of the heart.

Physical signs of the most usual valvular lesion of the heart.

The bicuspid valve is the commonest form of congenital valvular abnormality of aortic stenosis. Thephysical signs are:

1. On palpation, the apex beat is not normally shifted, and the character of the apex is a heavingapex bcat. A systolic thrill may be palpable.
2. On auscultation, an systolic ejection murmur is heard at the base, left sternal edge, aortic area,and carotids. Soft first heart sound. The second component of the second heart sound may be inaudible if the valve is calcified, and the second heart sound may be reversed due to the prolonged left ventricular ejection.

Question 152 Why is dyspnea caused by disorganization of the mitral valves?

Dyspnea caused by disorganization of the mitral valves Disorganization of the mitral valves willalter the hemodynamics of the cardiac output. In order that enough cardiac output to be maintained,the left atrial pressure increases, and left atrial hypertrophy and dilatation occurs. Consequently, the pulmonary venous, pulmonary arterial, and right heart pressures also increased. The development of pulmonary edema follows the increase in pulmonary capillary pressure. This is prevented by alveolar and capillary thickening and pulmonary arterial vasoconstriction. This would later lead to pulmonary hypertension, which causes right ventricular hypertrophy, dilatation, and failure. This pulmonary edema and heart failure will give rise to dyspnea.

Question 153 What are the physical signs of aortic regurgitation?

The pulse is bounding or collapsing. The apex beat is displaced laterally and is thrusting in nature. There is an early diastolic murmur at the left sternal edge. The other sign, which is rare,is due to the hyperdynamic circulation: Quincke's sign-capillary pulsation in the nail beds. De Musset's sign - head nodding with each heartbeat. Durozier's sign - Lightly applied systolic bruit over the femoral arteries with the stethoscope. The pistol shot the femoral - a sharp bang on auscultation over the femoral arteries with each heartbeat.

Question 154 Differentiate aortic and mitral valvular disease.

	Mitral stenosis	Mitral Regurgitation	Aortic stenosis	Aortic Regurgitation
Cause	Rheumatic heartdisease	Myxomatous degeneration infective endocardia subsvalvular dysfunction	Congenital bicuspid valve	Congenital bicuspid valve, infective endo carditis.

Palpation	Tapping apexbeat	Forceful apexbeat	Heaving apexbeat	Forceful and displaced apex beat
Auscultation	Loud first heartsound opening snap, mid-diastolic murmur	Pansystolic murmur, normalheart sound	Soft aortic component of second heart sound, ejection systolic murmur	Early diastolic murmur, normal heart sound

Question 155 Differentiate organic and functional heart murmurs.

	Functional murmur	Organic murmur
Timing	Systolic	Systolic and diastolic
Duration	Non-pansystolic	Can be the variable duration
Intensity	Grade 3 or less	Can be variable intensity
Radiation	Not wide	Can be variable radiation
Second heart sound	Normal respiratory variation	Normal respiratory variation
Evidence of heart disease	None	Yes

Question 156 Discuss the factors involved in selecting patients with mitral stenosis for commissurotomy

Factors involved in selecting patients with mitral stenosis for commissurotomy. 1. Uncontrollable pulmonary edema. 2. Limiting dyspnea and intermittent pulmonary edema.

3. Pulmonary hypertension with right ventricular hypertrophy or hemoptysis. 4. Limitationof activity despite ventricular rate control and medical therapy. 5. Recurrent systemic emboli despite anticoagulants with moderate or severe stenosis.

Question 157 List the common diagnostic errors associated with mitral stenosis

Common diagnostic errors associated with mitral stenosis. 1. Austin Flint murmur. 2. Left atrial myxoma. 3. Atrial septal defect (murmur originates in tricuspid valve area).
4. Ventricular septal defect or patent ductus arterious with the large left-right shunt. 5. Hypertrophic cardiomyopathy with left ventricular inflow tract obstruction. 6. Acute rheumatic mitral valvulitis (Carey Coomb murmur) 7. Constrictive pericarditis with involvement of the atrioventricular groove

Question 158 Describe the characteristics and significance of the several kinds of the arterial pulse.

Characteristics and significance of the several kinds of arterial pulse-

1. Small pulse volume - cardiac failure, hypovolemia, vasoconstriction.
2. Large volume pulse - vasodilatation. pyrexia, anemia, aortic regurgitation,arteriovenous shunting.
3. Pulse alternans an alternating pattern of large and small volume beats - cardiac failure
4. Pulsus paradoxus, the Systolic pressure falls

by 10 mm of Hg on inspiration -airways obstruction, pericardial tamponade, and massive pulmonary embolism.

5. Pulsus bisferiens. The first component is the clue to the percussion wave of a large volume of blood ejection in systole and the second component is due to elastic recoilin the arteries.

Question 159 Discuss the value or electrocardiography in the practice of medicine

Value of electrocardiography in the practice of medicine

Standard 12-lead Ecg - Used to elucidate cardiac arrhythmias and conduction defects, and diagnose and localize myocardial hypertrophy, ischemia, or infarction, provide informationabout electrolyte imbalance and certain toxicity of certain drugs.

Exercise stress ECG - Used for confirming a diagnosis of ischemic heart disease and to establish the severity and prognosis of ischemia heart disease_ It is indicated in

1. Screening an asymptomatic population for groups who E1.1-15 at high risk for coronary disease e.g., hyperlipidemic patients, and to study workers in critical positions military pilots.
2. For diagnostic evaluation of patients with chest pain not typical of angina pectoris

3. For evaluation of the degree of ischermia in patients with known angina or previous infarction about prognosis and treatment

4-evaluation therapeutic procedures in patients with angina e.g., coronary artery bypassgrafting, angioplasty, or trial of new drugs.

5. For evaluating the severity of other lesions, o_a. Aortic stenosis in children, mitral stenosis_

6. For evaluating work capacity e.g., following cardiac infarction.

7. For evaluating patients suspected of AY block or sinus node dysfunction.

C. Ambulatory ECG HOLTER MONITORING is used to detect transient episodes of- arrhythmia or ischemia., which seldom occur during the routine 12-lead ECG recordings.

Question 160 Give the formula of and show by the diagram, ventricular preponderance, or axis deviation.

The formula of ventricular axis deviation Lead I is positive, so the axis must be +30 degrees which are normal in left axis deviation. The main deflection is positive (R wave) in lead I and negative (S wave) in the lead III. In the right axis deviation, the main deflection is negative (S wave) ion lead I and positive (R wave) in lead III.

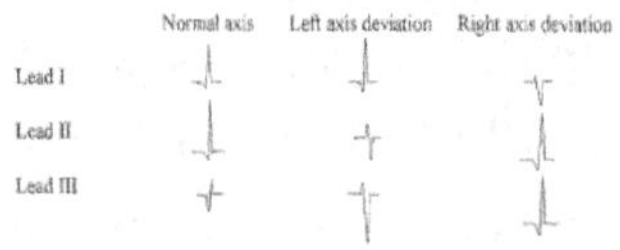

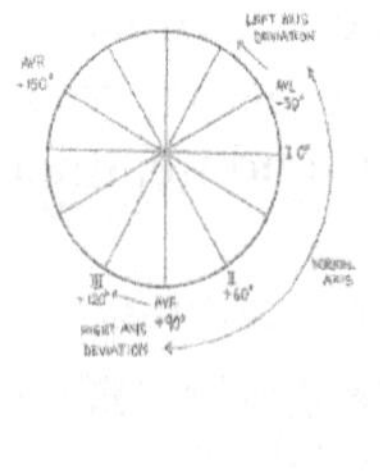

Question 161 What effects have large doses of digitalis had on the electrocardiogram?

Effects of large doses of digitalis on the electrocardiogram.
1. Bradycardia.
2. Multiple ventricular ectopic
3. Ventricular ligominy or alternate ventricular ectopic
4. Paroxysmal atrial tachycardia
5. Ventricular tachycardia
6. Ventricular fibrillation

Question 162 What changes occur in the electrocardiogram with abnormal potassium or calcium serum concentrations?

Electrocardiogram
1. Moderate hyperkalemia - Tall peaked T waves.
2. Severe hyperkalemia - Gross widening of the QRS with a resulting "sine wave appearance. P waves disappear
3. Hypokalemic - Prominent U waves with small T' waves resulting in an apparentlylong QT interval. T wave is often lost in the U wave.
4. Hypocalcemia - Long QT interval with small T waves
5. Hypocalcemia Short QT interval with normal T waves.

Question 163 Mention the significant diagnostic features of the electrocardiogram in a case of acute coronary occlusion with (a) anterior myocardial infarction and (b) posterior myocardial infarction.

6. Features of the electrocardiogram.

1. Small anterior - ST-segment elevation in V3-V4
2. Extensive anterior - ST-segment elevation in V2-VS
3. Anteroseptal - ST segment elevation in V1-V3
4. Anterolateral - ST-segment elevation, T wave inversion UI V4-V6, L, AVL

Posterior myocardial infraction.
Leads V1 and V2- initially tall R wave, St segment depression, and tell upright T waves.

Question 164 What special tests are sometimes employed in diagnosing heart disease?

Special tests are employed in the diagnosis of heart disease.
1. Exercise stress electrocardiography
2. Echocardiography - Transesophageal echocardiography and Doppler Echocardiography
3. Cardiac catheterization
4. Nuclear imaging – Thallium-201 imaging, pyrophosphate scan, radionuclideventriculography
5. CT scan and magnetic resonance imagining

Question 165 Discuss sinus tachycardia and sinus bradycardia briefly.

Sinus rate acceleration of more than 100

beats per minute is called sinus tachycardia

Causes.
1. Fever
2. Exercise
3. Emotion
4. Pregnancy
5. Anemia

6. Cardiac failure with compensatory sinus tachycardia.
7. Thyrotoxicosis
8. Catecholamines excess.
9. Primary sinus tachycardia

Treatment.

Correction of the underlying causes causing the tachycardia. Beta-blockers may beused to slow down the sinus rate if necessary.

Sinus bradycardia

A sinus rate of less than 60 beats per minute during the dayand less than 50 beats per minute at night is called sinus bradycardia. It is normal in athletes and in elderly patients. It is asymptomatic. The rate is very slow.

Causes

1. Hypothermia, hypothyroidism, cholestatic jaundice, and raised intracranial pressure
2. Drug therapy with beta-blockers, digitalis, and other antiarrhythmic drugs
3. Acute ischemia and infarction of the sinus node
4. Chronic degenerative changes such as fibrosis of the atrium ad sinus node

Treatment

Treatment of symptomatic sinus bradycardia is atropine 600 microgram intravenously.A cardiac pacemaker is required if symptomatic arrhythmia persists.

References

1. Harrison's Principles of Internal Medicine - 13th Edition,
2. Davidson's Principles and Practices of Medicine - 17th Edition.

Question 166 Define the various forms of cardiac

arrhythmia and briefly describe thedisturbance mechanism and the associated physical signs in the heart and pulse.

Cardiac arrhythmias.

A. Atrial tachyarrhythmias.

1. Atrial ectopic beats (extrasystole, premature beats). The ECG shows a premature hut otherwise normal ORS complex. It usually does not cause any symptoms, but it gives eSensation of a missed beat.

2. Arial tachycardia - It is due to increased automaticity or digitalis toxicity. The ECG shows an atrial rate of 140-220 per minute with abnormal P waves with variable AV blocks. It causes a sensation of palpation,

3. Atrial flutter. The ECG shows a rapid atrial rate of around 300 per minute with saw-toothed flutter waves and is associated with 2:1, 3:1, 4:1, or variable AV block; it causes a sensation of palpation

4.Atrial fibrillation - The atria beat rapidly and chaotically, and the ventricles respond at irregular intervals giving rise to an irregularly irregular pulse. The ECG shows normal but irregular ORS complexes with irregular fibrillation waves and noP waves.

B. Junctional tachyarrhythmias

I. AV nodal re-entry tachycardia - It is due to re-entry within the AV road and produces a regular tachycardia with a rate of 140-220 per minute. There is an awareness of palpation, and one feels faint or breathless. The ECG shows tachycardia withnormal QRS complexes

2 Wolff-Parkinson-White syndrome - There is an abnormal band of atrial tissue connecting the atria, ventricles, and car: electrically bypassing

the AV node. The ECG shows a shortening of the PR interval and a slurring of the QRS complex called a deltawave. It called paroxysms of tachycardia.

C. <u>Ventricular tachyarrhythmias</u>

1. Ventricular ectopic beats (extrasystoles, premature beats) - They can be found in normal people. It could manifest in patients with coronary heart disease, acute myocardial infarction, heart failure, mitral valve prolapses, and digoxin toxicity. The patientmay complain of an irregular heartbeat, missed beats, or abnormally strong beats, and irregular pulse with weak or missed beats.

2. Ventricular tachycardia - It is associated with serious heart disease and may degenerate into ventricular fibrillation. The ECG shows broad, abnormal QRS complex with a rate of 140-220 per minute. The patient may complain of palpitation,dizziness, dyspnea, or loss of consciousness.

3 Ventricular fibrillation. It is due to myocardial infarction, ischemia, or electrocution. The ECGshows chaotic, bizarre, irregular complexes. There is no pulse. The patient loses consciousness andcessation of respiration.

D. Sinoatrial disease (Sick Sinus Syndrome) is due to fibrosis, degenerative changes, or ischemia of the sinus node. The ECG shows intermittent tachycardia, bradycardia, or pauses withno atrial or ventricular activity,

E. Atrioventricular (AV) block.

1. First-degree AV block - The AV conduction is delayed, so the ECG shows thePR interval is prolonged longer than 0.20 seconds. There are no symptoms.

2. Second-degree AV block.

a. **Mobitz type 1 second degree** AV Mock-It is due to impaired conduction proximalto the bundle of his. Maybe due to physiological or in your young athlete with a high vagal tone. The ECG shows a progressive lengthening of successive PR intervals culminating in a dropped beat, and the cycle then repeats itself. The pulse will show amissed beat, and the patient may show faintness.

Mobitz type 2 second-degree AV block - It is due to diseases below the bundle ofhis, and symptoms are more serious than Mobitz type I. The FCG shows the PR interval remains constant, but some P waves are not conducted.

3. Third-degree (complete) AV block - It is when AV conduction fails completely, and te atria and ventricles beat independently; ventricular activity is maintained by an escape rhythm arising in the bundle of His (narrow QRS complexes) or the distal conducting tissues (broad QRS complexes). There will be a slow 25-50 per minute pulse, which does not vary with exercise. There may be a large volume pulse and systolic flow murmur due to a compensatory increase in stroke volume. Canon wavesmay be visible in the neck, and the intensity of the first heart sound varies due to the loss of AV synchrony.

4.Adams-Stokes attacks - It is when episodes of ventricular asystole complicate thecomplete heart block or Mobitz type Il second-degree AV block or in patients with Sino-atrial disease. There will be the sudden loss of consciousness which occur withoutwarning. Convulsions may occur due to cerebral ischemia if there is u prolonged asystole, and the recovery are rapid. There is pallor and a death-like appearance duringthe attack, but when the heart starts to beat again, there is a characteristic flush.

.

F. Bundle branch block and hemiblock - Il is due to the interruption of the right or leftbranch of the bundle of His due to conducting tissue diseases which delay the activation of the ventricles. The ECG shows a broadening of the ORS complexes (>0.12 seconds)

1. The right bundle branch block shows wide QRS complexes with an M-shapedconfiguration in leads VI and V2 and a wide S wave in the lead I
2. The left bundle branch block shows wide QRS complexes with loss of the Q wave in the lead I and M-shaped QRS complexes in V5 and V6.
3. Hemiblocks - The left branch of the bundle of His divides into anterior and posterior fascicles. Damage of the conducting tissue here does not broaden the QRS complex but alters the mean direction of ventricular depolarization, causing left axis deviation in the left anterior hemiblock and right axis deviation in the left posterior hemiblock.The combination of the right bundle branch block and the left anterior or posterior hemiblock is known as bifasciular block.

Question 167 What are the possible harmful effects of arrhythmia?

Harmful effects of arrhythmia the arrhythmia may cause sudden cardiac death, symptomatic syncope, near syncope, dizziness, or palpitations. It may also reduce the cardiac output so that thebrain's and the myocardium's perfusion is impaired or lead to a more serious arrhythmia withfatal consequences. Stable supraventricular tachycardia without underlying heart disease is generally well tolerated in most people but may lead to myocardial ischemia, congestive heart failure in patients with coronary heart disease, valvular abnormalities, and systolic or diastolic myocardial dysfunction. Ventricular tachycardia may degenerate into ventricular fibrillation, which is fatal if it is not cardio versed immediately. Bradycardia with complete heart block or transient standstill may produce syncope and convulsion.

Question 168 Outline the treatment for paroxysmal atrial tachycardia.

Treatment for paroxysmal atrial tachycardia

Mechanical measures of Valsalva 's maneuver and breath-holding - stimulate the vagus, which delay atrioventricular conduction and blocks the reentry mechanism, thus terminating the arrhythmias. Vagal stimulation with carotid sinus pressure over one carotid sinus for 10-20 seconds and then over the other carotid sinus.

Drug therapy

1. Intravenous adenosine, treatment of choice, 6 mg bolus dose and followed by a second and athird 12 mg bolus dose if there is no response.
2. Intravenous verapamil, 2.5 mg bolus, and another 2.5 mg to 5 mg every 1-3 minutes up to 20mg.
3. Intravenous esmolol, a short beta-blacker, 500 microgram/kg over 1 minute, followed by aninfusion of 25-200 microgram/minute.
4. Intravenous digoxin, 0.5-0_75 mg bolus, followed by 0.25 mg every 2-4 hours up to a total of1-1.25 mg.

Cardioversion is to be considered if the above drug therapy fails and if it warrants immediatetermination. Synchronized electrical cardioversion with 50-100 J.

Ablation of the atrioventricular node and the His bindle delivery of a high radio frequencyenergy to the atrioventricular node via a catheter eliminates the reentry circuit.

Pacemakers Programmed permanent pacemakers to sense the supraventricular tachycardia andpace to interrupt the reentry circuit and stop the arrhythmia.

Prophylactic drugs such as digoxin, verapamil, and sotalol.

Question 169 What is the significance of paroxysmal ventricular tachycardia, and what is the drugof choice in treatment?

Significance of paroxysmal ventricular tachycardia. It is usually a complication of acute myocardial infarction, dilated cardiomyopathy, mitral valve prolapses, myocarditis, hypertension, adcoronary artery disease. The drug of choice in treatment is amiodarone.

Question 170 What are the indications for converting atrial fibrillation to normal sine rhythm?

Indications for the conversion of atrial fibrillation to normal sinus rhythm

1. Immediate indications - hypotension, heart failure, and angina
2. Atrial fibrillation of recent onset (<12 months) and left atrial dilation are not severe.
3. Elective procedures following the first attack of atrial fibrillation with an identifiable cause - e.g.,pneumonia, a thoracotomy, pulmonary embolus, controlled thyrotoxicosis following thyroidectomy, coronary artery surgery, and mitral valve surgery.

Question 171 Give the causes and clinical picture of angina pectoris

Causes of angina pectoris

1. Coronary atheroma.
2. Fissured plaque with adherent thrombus.
3. Local coronary artery spasm.
4. 'Transient myocardial ischemia.
5. Aortic valve disease

6. Hypertrophic cardiomyopathy

The clinical picture of angina pectoris.
Left-sided or central chest pain precipitated by exertion, such as walking uphill, and relieved by rest and sublingual nitrate. Patients may describe the pain as tightness or heaviness onthe chest with the chest clenched fist and associated with breathlessness. Pain may radiate to the neck or jaw, with pain or heaviness radiating down the arms, usually on the left side. Sometimes, the pain can be in the epigastric or interscapular space. Physical signs are frequently negative.

Question 172 Describe the clinical picture and treatment of acute myocardial infarction

The clinical picture of acute myocardial infarction
The patient may present with chest pain, which is sudden in onset, occurring at rest, and lasting for a few hours. The chest pain can be very severe, and the patient may feel imminent doom or death, but it can also be less severe and arid, being mistaken for indigestion. The chest pain can be associatedwith sweating, nausea, -vomiting, restlessness, and anxiety. Some 20% of the patient may have apainless or silent myocardial infarction commonly seen in diabetics, hypertensives, and elderly patients, and they may present with breathlessness, hypotension, and arrhythmias

Physical signs - The patient may look pale, sweaty, and grey. Sinus tachycardia, hypotension, and abnormal precordial pulsation due to the systolic bulging of infracted myocardium, an additionalfourth heart sound, a raised venous pressure, and sad basal crackles. There may be a mild Fever due to muscle necrosis and a pericardial rub on auscultation.

Treatment of myocardial infarction
Patients should be managed in coronary care unit as soon as

possible.1 An intravenous
assessment for intravenous
fluids and medications.

2. Control pain of myocardial infarction. Diamorphine 5-10 mg intravenous and an emetic, suchas cyclizine 50 mg intravenous.

3. High flow of oxygen as the arterial PO2 is reduced in myocardial infarction. Oxygen at 60% isgiven by nasal cannula or face mask.

4. Oral aspirin of 300 mg in a soluble or chewable form and 150 mg daily may improve survival.

5. Fibrinolytic therapy reduces the mortality rate up to 301/a in the first 6 hours. a. Streptokinase 1.5 million units over 1 hour. b. Anistreplase - 30 units over5 minutes. c. Alteplase- 10 mgbrains, followed by 50 mg in the first hour, and 40 mg over the subsequent 2 hours.

6. Immediate coronary angioplasty if fibrinolytic therapy is contraindicated.

7. Anticoagulants - Subcutaneous heparin, 5000 units 8 hourly. Patients who received alteplasemust receive immediate heparin 10,000 units plus 1000 units hourly.

8. Beta-blockers - relieve pain, reduce arrhythmias, and improve short-term mortality in patients who present - within 12 hours of the onset of the symptoms. Intravenous atenolol 5-10 mg over 5 minutes or metoprolol 5 -15 mg over 5 minutes. It is contraindicated if patients havesevere bradycardia, heart failure, and heart block.

9. Nitrates Intravenous nitrates, nitroglycerin 0.6-1.2 mg/hour, or isosorbide dinitrate 1-2 mg/hourfor treatment of left ventricular failure and recurrent or persistent ischemic pain. Sublingual glyceryl trinitrate for persistent pain.

10. Bedrest for the first 24-48 hours with mild sedation if necessary and a quiet atmosphere

Question 173 What are the causes and treatment of palpitations of the heart?

Causes of palpitations of the heart

A. Non-cardiac lesions, e.g., exercise, thyrotoxicosis, anemia, anxiety, perimenopausalflushing, sudden vasodilatation following vasodilator drugs, alcohol, caffeine.
B. Cardiac lesions 1. Conditions that increase the stroke volume - regurgitant valvular diseases, bradycardia 2. Cardiac arrhythmias. a. Premature ectopic beats b. Paroxysmaltachycardia - paroxysmal atrial fibrillation, paroxysmal ventricular tachycardia. e.g., mitral valve disease, coronary artery disease, pericarditis, post-cardiac surgery, and recent myocardial infarction.

Treatment of palpitation

A. Non-cardiac lesions - treatment of the underlying conditions and reassurances. If necessary, a small dose of beta-blocker, such as propranolol, for symptomatic relief for thyrot oxicosis and anxiety.
B. Investigate the conditions which increase the stroke volume and treat the underlyinglesions.
C. Paroxysmal atrial fibrillation - No ideal treatment for this. Amiodarone may be useful iftreatment is needed.
D. D. Paroxysmal ventricular tachycardia - To treat the underlying cause. If it is needed, amiodarone may be used.

Question 174 Give the symptoms and signs of congestive heart failure. What are the general means of treatment?

Symptoms and signs of congestive heart failure. The clinical picture depends on the nature of the underlying causes. Generally, the patient may present with Fatigue, poor effort tolerance, andlistlessness in low output failure.

The peripheries are cold, and the blood pressure is low. Oliguria and uremia due to poor renal perfusion. Left heart failure may cause pulmonary edema presenting as breathlessness, orthopnea, paroxysmal nocturnal dyspnea, and inspiratory crackles over the basal lungs. Right heart failure produces a high jugular venous pressure with hepatic congestion and dependent edema, which may collect in the thighs and sacrum in a bed-bound patient. Massive accumulation of fluids may cause ascites or pleural effusion. Chronic heart failure may be associated with weight loss caused by anorexia and impaired gastrointestinal absorption due to gastrointestinal congestion, poor tissue perfusion due to low cardiac output, andskeletal muscle atrophy due to immobility.

Treatment.

A. Generally, the patient is advised for bed rest, which increases the renal blood flow andmay help in diuresis in a patient with severe heart failure. Later, the patient can do light exercises, walking, and swimming, which can improve the outlook of a patient with chronic heart failure. Patients should avoid high salt intake, excessive alcohol, and salt orfluid-retaining drugs.

B. B. Drug treatment.

1. Diuretics - reduce the preload and improve pulmonary and systemic venous congestion and may cause a fall in afterload and ventricular volume leading to a fallin wall tension and increased cardiac efficiency. Diuretics, such as loop diuretics - frusemide and bumetanide, thiazide diuretics - bendrofluazide, potassium-sparing diuretics - spironolactone. In severe heart failure, the combination of different diuretics (loop, thiazide, and potassium-sparing) may increase the diuretic effect and help to prevent hypokalemia.

2. Angiotensin-converting enzyme inhibitors - They prevent the conversion of angiotensin I to angiotensin II, thus counteracting salt and water retention, peripheralarterial and venous vasoconstriction, and activation of the sympathetic nervous system.
Therefore, a reduction in the afterload. Captopril 25 mg 8 hourly, enalapril 20 mg daily, and lisinopril 10 mg daily are used. The combination of a potassium-losing diuretic and an ACE inhibitor may have potential advantages.
3. Digoxin - used in the patient with heart failure and atrial fibrillation to provide control of the ventricular rate and a small positive inotropic effect.

C. Cardiac transplantation. Treatment of choice in younger patients with severe, intractable heart failure whose life expectancy is less than 6 months, some patientswith coronary artery disease and dilated cardiomyopathy.

Question 175 Define and give a classification of hypertension.

Hypertension. The World Health Organization has defined hypertension as blood pressure measurement higher than 160/95 mmHg. The Framingham Study defined 160/95 mmHg as abnormal and 140/90 to 160/95 mmHg as borderline hypertension.

Classification of hypertension. Essential hypertension 1. Genetic and familial factors.
2. Socioeconomic - related to social deprivation. 3. Environmental factors. 4.

Dietaryfactors - obesity, high alcohol, high salt intake, caffeine. 5. Hormonal factors - highrenin, reduced nitric oxide, atrial natriuretic peptide, anti-diuretic hormone effects. 6.Neurotransmitters - acetylcholine, norepinephrine, substance P, neuropeptide Y, serotonin, dopamine, encephalin.

B. Secondary hypertension

1. Renal causes., E.g., glomerulonephritis, chronic pyelonephritis, collagen vascular disease.

b. Polycystic kidney disease. c. renal artery stenosis.

2. Coarctation of the aorta

3. Endocrine causes a. Pheochromocytoma b. Cushing's syndrome. c. Conn's syndrome (primary hyperaldosteronism) d. Hyperparathyroidism. e. Acromegaly. f. Primary hypothyroidism. g. Congenital adrenal hyperplasia. h. 11 beta-hydroxylase, 17-hydroxylasedeficiency.

4. Drugs. E.g., Oral contraceptives containing estrogens, anabolic steroids, corticosteroids,non-steroidal anti-inflammatory drugs, carbenoxolone, and sympathomimetic agents.

5. Pregnancy - pre-eclampsia or toxemia of pregnancy.

Question 176 *D*ifferentiate benign from malignant hypertension.

Malignant hypertension: It presents with visual impairment, nausea, vomiting, fits, transientparalysis, several headaches, impairment of consciousness, or symptoms of acute cardiac failure.

Benign hypertension: There is high blood pressure,

but usually there are no abnormal signs,symptoms, or abnormal investigation.

Question 177 Discuss the treatment of essential hypertension.

Treatment of essential hypertension. Persistent systolic pressure above 160 mmHg shouldbe treated with the aim of reducing it to about 150/95 mmHg.

General measure. 1. Weight reduction. 2. Restriction of excessive intake of alcohol and saltand stop smoking. 3. Regular exercise and meditation - to reduce anxiety and stress. 4.
Correct hyperlipidemia to reduce the risk of atheroma.

B. Drugs. 1. Diuretics - Lower the blood pressure by sodium and water excretion and dilating the arterioles. Loop diuretics e.g., frusemide 40 mg daily or bumetanide 1-2 mg daily, thiazide diuretics e.g., bendrofluazide 5 mg daily or cyclopenthiazide 0.5 mg daily. 2. Beta-blockers - Their mechanism of action is not clear. It may act by reducing the force of cardiac contraction and renin production. Propranolol 80 mg twice daily, atenolol 50-100 mgdaily, and oxprenolol 80 mg daily. Cardio-selective beta-blockers, such as atenolol and metoprolol.

3. Calcium antagonists - Reduce the blood pressure by arteriolar dilatation and reducingthe force of contraction. Nifedipine 20 mg twice daily, diltiazem 60 mg three times daily, verapamil 120-240 mg daily

in divided doses, and amlodipine 5-10 mg once daily.

Angiotensin-converting enzyme (ACE) inhibitors - Blocks the conversion of angiotensin Ito angiotensin II, a powerful vasoconstrictor. Captopril 50-150 mg daily in divided doses, lisinopril 10-20 mg daily, and enalapril 10 20 mg daily.

If the general measure to control hypertension fails to reduce the high blood pressure diureticor a beta-blocker is prescribed. Diuretics are preferred, e.g., bendrofluazide 5-10 mg daily if there is heart failure or a peripheral disease is present. Beta-blockers are used if the patient also has angina. If a single drug does not work, then the diuretics can be combined with a beta-blocker or a calcium antagonist if these prove inadequate, then ACE inhibitors may be used, especially if the patient has associated diabetes. Patient education is important as the treatment is for many years or life.

Question 178 Discuss the significance of myocarditis

Myocarditis - The most common form of the inflammatory endomyocardial disease is myocarditis.It can be due to idiopathic or infective etiology.

Causes. 1. Viruses - e.g., Coxsackie, influenza, rubella, polio, adenovirus, echovirus. 2. Protozoa - e.g., Trypanosoma cruzi, toxoplasma gondii. 3. Radiation, chemicals, drugs - e.g.,lead poisoning, emetine, and chloroquine. 4. Bacterial infection - e.g., Corynebacterium, Rickettsia, Chlamydia, and

Coxiella.

Clinical features. It usually presents as an acute illness with fever and cardiac failure. In addition, there maybe a history of respiratory or febrile illness. Physical cardiovascular signs are a soft heartsound, a loud third heart sound, tachycardia, and sometimes, a friction rub.

Investigations. 1. Chest X-ray – may show an enlarged cardiac shadow. 2. ECG – may showST and T wave abnormalities and arrhythmias. 3. Elevated cardiac enzymes and viral antibody titers may be raised, and cardiac biopsy may show inflammation

Treatment Bed rest and eradication of any acute infection. Treatment of cardiac failure and cardiac arrhythmias. The prognosis is usually good, but chronic cardiomyopathy may develop.

Question 179 Differentiate a pericardial friction sound from pleurisy without effusion.

Pericardial friction sound	Pleurisy without effusion
It is relieved by sitting forward	No relieving position
It is aggravated by lying down and movement	It is aggravated by deep inspiration coughing with twisting and bending movement

High-pitched superficial scratching sound caused by movement of the inflamed pericardium. Best heard with both held inspiration and expiration on auscultation	A plural rub is heard during deep inspiration and expiration on auscultation
Causes: - Coxsackie viral infection, myocardial infarction, uremia, connective tissue disease, tuberculosis, and malignancy.	Pneumonia, pulmonary infarct malignancy, rheumatoid arthritis, systemic lupus erythematosus

Qucstion 180 What are the symptoms and signs of (a) acute fibrinous pericarditis, (b)pericarditis with effusion (c) chronic constrictive pericarditis?

Acute fibrinous pericarditis. The pain of pericarditis is retrosternal and radiates to the shoulders and neck and is aggravated by deep inspiration, movement, a change of position,exercise, and swallowing. There may be a pericardial rub which is high pitched superficial scratching noise produced by the movement of the inflamed pericardium and is diagnostic of pericarditis. The rub is detectable on auscultation in held inspiration and expiration.

Pericarditis with effusion. There may be a sensation of retrosternal oppression. The physical signs are difficult in eliciting. The heart sound may be soft, and no pericardial rub is heard.

Chronic constrictive pericarditis. There will be signs and symptoms of systemic venous congestion indicative of constrictive pericarditis. There may be right heart failure, hepatomegaly, ascites, and atrial fibrillation. There may be mild breathlessness as the lungsare not congested.

Question 181 Make a diagnosis of an aneurysm of the descending aorta.

Diagnosis of aneurysm of the descending aorta. Diagnosis is suggested by the presence of an acute onset of severe pain in the chest or between the shoulder blades. There may be hypertension and asymmetry of the brachial, carotid, or femoral pulses. The patient will be in shock and inappropriate bradycardia from stimulation of aortic baroreceptors. Chest X-rayshows a widened mediastinum a left pleural effusion. CT scan and transesophageal echocardiography are diagnostic. Angiography is needed if the above investigation is inconclusive.

Question 182 Make a diagnosis of an aneurysm of the descending aorta.

Diagnosis of aneurysm of the descending aorta. Diagnosis is suggested by the presence of anacute onset of severe pain in the chest or between the shoulder blades. There may be hypertension and asymmetry of the brachial, carotid, or femoral pulses. The patient will be in shock and inappropriate bradycardia from stimulation of aortic baroreceptors. Chest X-rayshows a widened mediastinum a left pleural effusion. CT scan and transesophageal echocardiography are diagnostic. Angiography is needed if the above investigation is inconclusive.

Clinical picture. The clinical picture is related to the pulmonary disorder and is presented as chronic productive cough, exertional dyspnea, wheezing respiration, easy fatigability, and weakness. When right heart failure occurs due to pulmonary disorder, there may bedependent edema and right upper quadrant pain. The physical signs of cor pulmonale are cyanosis, clubbing, distended neck veins, right ventricular heave epigastric pulsation, an enlarged liver, and dependent edema.

Treatment Vigorous therapy of the pulmonary disorder responsible for right heart failure may lead to marked improvement of blood gases and improvement of heart failure.Acute chest infections must be treated. Oxygen therapy over a period may reduce established pulmonary hypertension. Extensive surgical removal of organized thrombus may be needed.

Question 183 What factors play a role in peripheral vascular disease?

Factors which a role in peripheral vascular disease.

1. Arteriosclerosis - This is an age-related arterial change with compensatory muscular hypertrophy of the media, followed by fibrosis and dilatation of the lumen.

2. Monckeberg ‘s sclerosis - It is commonly seen in the major lower arteries of the elderly and the diabetic arterial vessel. This degenerative disease ofunknown cause is characterized by dystrophic calcification of the media.

3. Cystic medial necrosis or degeneration - This is the mucoid degenerationof the collagen and the elastic tissue of the media. It is seen commonly in elderly hypertensives.

4. Atheroma - This is due to atheromatous degeneration of the vessel.

Question 184 Differentiate between intermittent claudication and rest pain.

Intermittent claudication

This ischemic, cramp-like pain usually in the calves during exercise and relieved by rest and is seen in occlusive arterial disease.

Rest pain

This is the continuous burning pain due to ischemia of the lower leg, whichbegins or is aggravated after reclining and is relieved by sitting or standing.

Question 185 Differentiate between gangrene due to arteriosclerosis, thromboangiitis obliterans (Buerger's disease), and Raynaud disease.

Gangrene due to arteriosclerosis.

The peripheral limb will be cold with dry skin, lack of hair, and absence of pulses todiseased areas. X-ray of the limbs may show calcification of the arteries.

Gangrene due to thromboangiitis (Buerger's disease).

This involves the lower limb's small vessels, which occur in young men who smoke. There is an inflammatory reaction in the arterial wall with the involvement of the neighboring vein and nerve, terminating in the thrombosis of the artery. There initially was peripheral ischemia with cold limbs and severe pain. The gangrene starts in the digits, commencing inthe distal portion of the digit near the nail and gradually extending proximally to involve the whole foot or hand.

Gangrene due to Raynaud's disease.

This is commonly seen in females. It usually affects the tip of the finger, which starts withulceration due to obstruction and not due to spasms of the arterioles. The fingers graduallybecome wasted, especially at the pulps, which become thin and pointed. Small and painfulischemic ulcers may be seen on the fingertips. The patient gradually gets rest pain and gangrene of the fingertips.

Question 186 Outline the treatment for motion sickness (air or sea sickness).

1. Light meals of easily digested food before and during the flight may reduce the tendencyto nausea and vomiting.
2. Sedatives or antihistamines before and during flight. Eg. dimenhydrinate 50 mg everyhour, promethazine 25 mg every 6 hours, or meclizine 25-50 mg every 24 hours.
3. One transdermal scopolamine disk was applied behind one ear at least 4 hours before the journey.

Question 187 What is the significance of thrombophlebitis in relation to malignant lesions?

Significance of thrombophlebitis in relation to malignant lesions. Malignancy causes hypercoagulability condition, which results in the formation of venous thrombi consisting of red cells, fibrin, and platelets which may embolize the deep veins of the leg and causethrombophlebitis.

Question 188 Outline the management of a case of electric shock.

Management of a case of electric shock

A. Urgent measures. Patients with electrical shock are to be kept away from the source ofthe current with precautions taken for the rescuer. Cardiopulmonary support must be initiated immediately, as the patient can be resuscitated successfully without neurological damage, even after a prolonged cessation of vital functions.

B. Hospital management.

1 Intravenous fluid replacement is very important as fluid is rapidly lost into damaged tissues. Failure to correct the hypovolemia will result in acute renal failure. Normalsaline should be infused rapidly at 0.5-1 ml/kg/hour to correct hypo vole to maintain urine output with a minimum of 100 mL/hour. Red blood cell transfusion, fresh frozen plasma, or plasma expander are not needed in the acute resuscitation phase.

2 Observation to prevent shock, hemorrhage, thrombosis, and myoglobinuria. Electrocardiography is to observe for arrhythmias, infarction, and echocardiography forsudden cardiac dilation, which may be fatal to the patients.

3 Evaluation for blunt injuries like fractures, skin burns from the entry and exit wound fromthe electrical shock, neurologic damage, and acid-base disturbances.

4 The aim is to stabilize the patient, salvage the limb debridement of devitalized tissues,wound coverage, and rehabilitation.

5 Prophylactic antibiotics, such as aqueous penicillin the given till proper identification ofthe organism. Burn wounds sustained can be covered with silver sulfadiazine cream or sulfamoyl cream. Commonly, coverage of open wounds usually requires skin grafting.

6 Good nutrition support and physiotherapy with splints and an aggressive program of physical therapy for the patients.

7 Psychological counseling for patients who have to require major amputation or other surgical procedures.

Question 189 Differentiate between heat exhaustion, heat stroke, and heat cramp.

Heat exhaustion. It is caused by water depletion or salt and water depletion due to sweating.It is seen in the person who is not acclimatized to hot climates and undertakes heavy exercise. Water loss can be as high as 5-6 liters per day, and up to 20 g of salt can be lost. They maypresent as giddiness, generalized fatigue, weakness, syncope, hypotension, raised body temperature to 38-40 degrees Celsius, signs of volume depletion, dehydration, and delirium.

Heat stroke. It is a life-threatening condition where the body temperature is above 41 degrees Celsius. The person is usually unacclimated to hot and humid climates. Heatstroke can occur without exercise, and there is no sweating. The person presents with headache, nausea, vomiting, weakness, skin is hot, and leading to confusion and delirium coma.

Heat cramp. It is caused by low extracellular sodium caused by replenishing water butnot salt during prolonged sweating. The person presents with painful cramps in the leg muscles after exercise. This condition often occurs in fit young persons who are well acclimatized when they exercise heavily in hot weather.

Question 190 Discuss long-term anticoagulant therapy.

Long-term anticoagulant therapy

For long-term use of anticoagulant, coumarin_ warfarin is ideal as it has a low incidence of side effects other than bleeding. Warfarin dosages are calculated based on the internationalnormalized ratio (INR), which is the ratio of the patient's PT (prothrombin time) to a normalcontrol when using the international reference preparation.

Identification of anticoagulant therapy based on the INR therapeutic ranges

A. INR of 2.0-3.0. Treatment for: 1. Deep vein thrombosis, pulmonary embolism, and systemic embolism. 2. Transient ischemic attack, 3. Atrial fibrillation, 4. Mitral stenosis with embolism.
B. B. INR of 3,0-4,5.
   Treatment for: 1.

Recurrent deep venous thrombosis and pulmonary embolism. 2. Arterial disease, including myocardial infarction. 3. Arterial grafts. 4. Cardiac prosthetic valves and grafts.

C. Contraindications to the use of warfarin 1. Severe hypertension. 2. Non-thrombo-embolic strokes. 3. Peptic ulceration. 4. Severe liver and renal disease. 5. Pre-existing hemostatic defects. 6. Pregnancy - warfarin is teratogenic in the first trimester, and fetal hemorrhage may occur later in the pregnancy.

Clinical conditions which affect the response to warfarin

A. An effect of increased anticoagulation due to warfarin. 1. Drugs were causing a reduction inthe metabolism of warfarin. e.g., tricyclic antidepressants, cimetidine, sulphonamides, phenothiazines, and amiodarone. 2. Drugs that increase the sensitivity of hepatic receptors to warfarin. e.g., clofibrate, quinidine. 3. Drugs interfering with vitamin K absorption may potentiate the action of warfarin e.g., broad-spectrum antibiotics and cholestyramine. 4. The displacement of warfarin from its binding site on serum albumin, e.g., sulphonamides. 5. Drugs that inhibit platelet function will increase the risk ofbleeding. e.g., aspirin. 6. Alcohol excess, cardiac failure, liver or renal disease, thyrotoxicosis, and febrile illness may potentiate the effect of warfarin.

B. An effect of decreased anticoagulation due to warfarin. 1. Drugs that increase the clearance of warfarin by induction of hepatic enzymes that metabolize warfarin. rifampicin,barbiturates. 2. Hypothyroidism 3. Transfusion of whole blood or fresh frozen plasma. 4.
Diet high in vitamin K (green vegetables) 5. Hereditary warfarin resistance.

Management of over-coagulation with warfarin 1. Life-threatening hemorrhage - Give vitamin K 5 mg by slow intravenous infusion and fresh frozen plasma orconcentrates of factor II, IX, and X with frozen VII concentrate. 2. Less severe hemorrhage - withhold warfarin for one or two days and consider giving vitamin K 0.5-2 mg intravenously. 3. INR of >4.5 without hemorrhage - withdraw warfarin for 1 to 2 days andthen review. 4. Unexpected bleeding at therapeutic ranges - investigate the possibility of the underlying cause, such as renal or alimentary tract disease.

References

1. Harrison 's Principles of Internal Medicine -13th Edition.
2. Davidson 's Principles and Practices of Medicine – 17th Edition

Question 191 Give classification of kidney disease

Classification of kidney disease

A. Congenital abnormalities of the kidneys. 1. Polycystic kidney disease. 2. Medullary cysticdisease and medullary sponge kidney. 3. Agenesis, hypoplasia, ectopic kidneys. 4. Alport's syndrome, congenital nephrotic syndrome, renal tubular transport defects, and renal glycosuria.

B. Tumors of the kidney. 1. Malignant renal tumors - renal cell carcinoma, nephroblastoma(Wilm's tumor). 2. Benign renal tumors - renal adenoma, simple cysts.

C. Glomerular disease. 1. Glomerulonephritis - a. Proliferative glomerulonephritis - diffuseproliferative glomerulonephritis, focal segmental glomerulonephritis, crescentic glomerulonephritis, mesangiocapillary glomerulonephritis. b. Membranous glomerulonephritis. c. Minimal change glomerular lesion, d. IgA nephropathy. e. Henoch-Schoenlein syndrome, f. Focal segmental glomerulosclerosis. 2. Acute nephritic syndrome. 3.Goodpasture's syndrome

D. Kidney in systemic disease. 1. Systemic vasculitis - Systemic lupus erythematosus, Systemic vasculitis - polyarteritis nodosa, microscopic polyarteritis, Wegener's granulomatous. 2. Others - diabetes mellitus, systemic sclerosis, amyloidosis, hemolyticuremic syndrome, thrombotic thrombocytopenic purpura, multiple myeloma, contrast nephropathy, hypertension, hyperuricemia nephropathy

E. Major manifestations of renal disease - are nephrotic syndrome, and acute and chronic renal failure.

F. Infection of kidney and urinary tract –

infection of the upper and lower urinary tractG.

Renal calculi and nephrocalcinosis

H. Urinary tract infection

I. Drug-induced renal disease – 1. drug-induced

tubular necrosis 2. Acute ischemic tubularnecrosis. 3. Acute tubulointerstitial nephritis. 4. Obstruction – retroperitoneal fibrosis, crystals. 5. Papillary necrosis and chronic interstitial nephritis.

Question 192 Define hydronephrosis. State its cause and describe its treatment.

Hydronephrosis Dilation of the renal pelvis due to obstruction at any point b/w the kidneyand the urethral meatus

Causes.

A Within the lumen 1. Calculus and blood clots 2. Sloughed papilla due to diabetes, analgesic abuse, sickle cell disease, or trait 3. Tumor of the renal pelvis or ureter and bladdertumor.

B Within the wall 1. Pelviureteric neuromuscular dysfunction (congenital. 10% bilateral) 2.Ureteric stricture tuberculosis, especially after treatment; calculus, after Surgery) 3.
Ureterovesical structure (congenital, ureterocele; calculus; schistosomiasis) 4. Congenital megaureter, congenital bladder neck obstruction. 5. Neuropathic bladder. 6. Urethral stricture (calculus, gonococcal: after instrumentation) 7. Congenital urethral valve and pin-hole meatus

C Pressure from outside. 1. Pelviureteric compression (bands, aberrant vessels) 2. Tumors (e.g., retroperitoneal tumor or glands, carcinoma of the colon) 3. Diverticulitis, aortic aneurysm, retroperitoneal fibrosis, accidental ligation of the ureter, retrocaval ureter, prostatic obstruction, phimosis. 4. Tumors in the pelvis (e.g., cervix carcinoma).

Treatment Aim of treatment is to preserve renal function and to relieve the symptoms,

A. Relieving the obstruction. External drainage of urine by nephrostomy, and insertion of stentsto relieve obstruction, either temporary or permanent, are used to preserve the renal function, allow time for investigation, or when immediate surgery is hazardous.

B. Treating the Underlying causes.

C. Preventing or Treating the Infection.

D. Surgery. Nephrectomy or nephroureterectomy is used if the obstruction is due to malignant disease or the renal excretory function will return after relief of the obstruction. Permanent urinary diversion is required if the obstruction cannot be relieved. Ureteric anastomosis to an ileal conduit opening onto the abdominal wall is a method of diversion. Insertion of an indwelling catheter or stent into a ureter can relieve the obstruction of somepatients. A high obstruction in the urinary tract may require a permanent nephrostomy.

Question 193 Describe pyuria and state its importance

Pyuria - The presence of more than five leukocytes per high-power field is considered significant pyuria.

Importance of pyuria - The presence of pyuria indicates injury to the urinary tract, whichmay or may not be due to infection. Pyuria may also be seen in the calculous disease, stricture disease, neoplasm, glomerulonephropathy and interstitial cystitis.

Question 194 What is the practical importance of hematuria, And How can its source bediagnosed?

Importance of hematuria. Blood in the urine is called hematuria. The presence of red cell casts indicates a glomerular lesion. Red cells which are deformed and cremated indicate upper urinary tract infection. Red cells with normal morphology indicate ureteric, bladder, prostatic or urethral bleeding.

Hematuria is diagnosed - Through a combination of patient history, physical examination, urinalysis, and often further diagnostic tests. A urinalysis is the initial step, involving the microscopic examination of a urine sample for red blood cells. Imaging studies such as ultrasound or CT scans, as well as blood tests, may be employed to identify the source and cause of the hematuria. The diagnostic approach is tailored to the individual's symptoms, medical history, and clinical findings to determine the underlying condition necessitating appropriate treatment.

Urinalysis and urine culture - Red cell casts and proteinuria suggest renal origin. Positive culture, bacteria, and irritating voiding symptoms in females suggest urinary tractinfection.

2. Cytology - assist in the diagnosis of neoplasms.

3. Upper tract imaging - may identify neoplasms of the kidney or ureter and benign lesions,such as urolithiasis and obstructive uropathy. Papillary

necrosis, medullary sponge kidney, or polycystic kidney disease.

4. Cystoscopy - assess for bladder or urethral neoplasm, benign prostatic enlargement, and radiation or chemical cystitis.

Question 195 Give the signs and symptoms of the floating kidney.

Floating kidney A hypermobile kidney is called a floating kidney.

Signs and symptoms. A palpable kidney may be palpable by abdominal palpation. Thepatient may present with a vague loin or abdominal discomfort. It may be related to impaired urinary drainage with secondary obstruction or stone formation.

Question 196 Make a differential diagnosis between renal colic and hepatic colic.

Renal colic - It is a pain due to thrombosis of the renal vein or artery, dissection of the renal artery, renal infarction, interareal mass lesions, or passage of a stone within the collecting system.

Hepatic colic - It is a pain due to the passage of the gallstones along the bile duct.

Question 197 Describe and give the significance of the various pathways of development of urinary tract infections.

Urinary tract infections (UTI)

A UTI is often due to bacteria from the patient's own bowel flora. B. Transfer to the urinary tract can beby the bloodstream, the lymphatics, by direct Extension, e.g., from a vesicocolic fistula, or via the ascendingtransurethral route C. UTI from the ascending transurethral route can be transmitted by 1. The paraurethral region is heavily colonized with bacteria thus increasing the risk of UTL. The other factorsinvolved are previous UTI, gross lack of personal hygiene, wearing nappies or sanitary towels, and local infection, e.g., vaginitis 2. Bacteria are transferred along the urethra to the bladder, which can be transmitted by catheterization or sexual intercourse. 3. Establishment and multiplication of bacteria within the bladder. A poor flow rate and infrequent and poor bladder emptying can predispose to infection.

Question 198 What is the significance of pyelonephritis?

Significance of pyelonephritis. Pyelonephritis is due to infection of the renal parenchyma due to ascending of organisms by the ureter and sometimes via blood borne. It can be caused by bacteria, suchas E coli, Proteus species, Klebsiella, Staphylococci or streptococci, or virulent organisms. The presence of complications may increase the risk of pyelonephritis, such as:

1. Abnormal urinary tract, e.g., obstruction, calculi, vesicoureteric reflux, neurological abnormality,indwelling catheter, chronic prostatitis, cystic kidney, analgesic nephropathy, renal scarring

2. Impaired renal function.

3. The associated disorder impairs defense mechanisms, e.g., diabetes, immunosuppressive therapy. Stasis within the tract compromises its defenses, and renal cysts and medullary scars due to previous inflammation facilitate the establishment of bacteria because they obstruct groups of nephrons. Once the infection is

established, eradication is difficult because the low blood flow, high osmolality, and high concentration of hydrogen ions and ammonia interfere with the mobilization of leukocytes and phagocytosis.

Question 199 What is the significance of persistent or recurrent urinary tract infections?

Significance of persistent or treat infections of the urinary tract.

Persistent urinary tract infections show that there is a source of persistent infection in contact withthe urinary tract. This may result from infected stones, chronic pyelonephritis, or prostatitis, vasicentric or vesicovaginal fistulae, obstructive uropathy, foreign bodies, or urethral diverticula.

Question 200 Give antimicrobial therapy for acute pyelonephritis.

Antimicrobial therapy of acute pyelonephritis. A. Mild symptoms. Symptomatic treatment with a potassium citrate mixture of 10 ml three times daily can be given pending the urinary culture results. B. Severe symptoms. Treatment for 3 to 5 days of Amoxycillin 250 mg three times daily, nitrofurantoin 50 mg three times daily, or trimethoprim 200 mg twice daily should be started immediately without waiting for the urinary culture results. A high volume of fluid intake, 2 liters, should be encouraged during treatment and subsequently C. If the patient is severely ill with high fever, loin pain, and tenderness: Intravenous ampicillin or Amoxycillin 1 gram 6 hourly or gentamicin2-5 mg/kg daily in divided doses should be given and switching to a further 7 days oral treatment when symptoms improve. Intravenous fluids to achieve good urinary output.

Question 201 Define pneumaturia.

Pneumaturia is the presence of gas in the urine, secondary to a fistula b/w bladder and the gastrointestinal tract. The other causes are diverticulitis, carcinoma of the bladder or sigmoid colon,and regional enteritis.

Question 202 What is the significance of pyuria with sterile urine cultures?

The significance of pyuria with sterile urine cultures is. Pyuria, which depends on the leukocyte countcan vary depending on the state of hydration, method of collection, and the degree of injury to the urinary tract. The other conditions where pyuria exists with sterile urine cultures are interstitial cystitis, calculous disease, stricture disease, neoplasm, or glomerulonephropathy,

Question 203 What is meant by renal glycosuria?

Renal glycosuria is when there is glucose in the urine of a patient who has normal blood glucose. It can be due to a defect in the tubular threshold for the reabsorption of glucose in the proximal tubule or a defect in the maximal tubular reabsorption of glucose.

Question 204 Discuss the etiology of impotence.

Etiology of Impotence Many patients with impotence have no definable organic cause. *A* careful history of physical disease, related symptoms, stress, and psychological factors, together with drugand alcohol abuse, must be taken. The presence of nocturnal emission and frequent satisfactory morning erections largely excludes endocrine disease as a cause. Psychological impotence is frequently a diagnosis of exclusion. The following are some of the important causes of impotence.

A. Psychological

B. Neurological

C. Vascular disease involving the pudendal artery and its branches,

D. Endocrine cause. 1. Reduced gonadotrophins. a. Hyperprolactinemia b Selective gonadotrophin deficiency - Kalman 's syndrome 2. Hyperprolactinemia 3. Congenital gonadal disease. 2. Anarchical/Leydig cell agenesis b. Chromosomal abnormality - e.g., Klinefelter's syndrome c. Enzyme defects 4. Acquired gonadal disease a. Testicular torsion b. Castration c. Local testicular disease. d. Chemotherapy and radiation toxicity, e. Rena failure f. Cirrhosis due toalcohol g. Sickle-cell disease 5. Androgen receptor deficiency 6. Systemic cases - Diabetes, hyperthyroidism, Addison's disease, acromegaly, multiple sclerosis, and tabes dorsalis.

E. Drug-induced 1. Alcohol 2. Cannabis 3. Beta-blockers 4. Diuretics 5. Metoclopramide 6. Methyldopa

Question 205 Describe the clinical features of acute glomerulonephritis

Clinical features of acute glomerulonephritis. The majority of the patients may present with unselective proteinuria, which may be enough to cause the nephrotic syndrome. Peripheral edema may develop if plasma albumin concentration is below 3 grams/dL, and may be associated withexertional dyspnea, pleural effusions, or ascites. Hematuria is present, and the presence of red cell casts are diagnostic of glomerular bleeding. Mainly, the patient's renal function is normal, butsome may develop significant impairment of function, and a small proportion proceeds to chronicrenal failure. A proportion of the patients will develop hypertension.

Question 206 Enumerate the points of value in the diagnosis of a case of chronic glomerulonephritis.

Diagnosis of chronic glomerulonephritis.

1. Patient presenting with persistent urinary abnormalities e.g., proteinuria or hematuria, and by slowly progressive impairment of renal function, eventuating in hypertension, contracted, granular kidneys, and end-stage renal failure.

2. Screening of asymptomatic patients with incidental findings of abnormal urine, impaired renalfunction, or hypertension. 3. Patients with insidious onset of symptoms and signs of renal disease,especially anemia and hypertension. 4. Patients with the previous history of viral or bacterial infection manifesting signs and symptoms of chronic glomerulonephritis.

Question 207 Give the indications for dialysis (artificial kidney) in treating uremia.

Indications for dialysis in the treatment of uremia. 1. Increased plasma levels of urea or creatinine concentration. A plasma level of urea greater than 30 mmol/L and creatinine greaterthan 600 micromole/L. 2. Hyperkalemia. 3. Fluid overload is not controlled by fluid restriction and diuretics. 4. Uremic pericarditis.

Question 208 Define and give a classification of

uremia.

Uremia. It is the excess nitrogenous end-product of protein and amino acid metabolism in theblood.

Classification of uremia.

A. Renal perfusion. 1. Arterial hypotension - e.g., gastrointestinal bleeding. 2. Decreased systemic vascular resistance - e.g., sepsis. 3. Defective renal autoregulation - e.g., ACE inhibitorsand NSAIDs. 4. Hepatorenal syndrome.

B. Renal vasculature. 1. Renal artery stenosis. 2. Renal embolism. 3. Renal arterioles - polyarteritis nodosa and accelerated hypertension. 4. Glomerular capillaries - Goodpasture's syndrome, Wegener's diseases, microscopic polyarteritis, pre-eclampsia, hemolytic uremicsyndrome, and cholesterol embolism. 5. Renal vein thrombosis.

C. Glomerulonephritis.

D. Tubules 1. Interstitial nephritis. 2. Drug-induced nephropathy - e.g., corticosteroids, tetracycline. 3. Contrast nephropathy. 4. Urate nephropathy. 5. Acute tubular necrosis.

Question 209 Give the causes, clinical picture, and treatment of the nephrotic syndrome.

Causes of nephrotic syndrome. 1. All glomerulonephrites and minimal-change glomerular lesions. 2. Systemic vasculitides, such as systemic lupus erythematosus. 3. Diabetic glomerulosclerosis. 4. Amyloidosis. 5. Drugs-e.g., penicillamine 6. Allergies - e.g., poison ivy.pollens, bee stings.

Clinical picture. The patient may notice that the urine is frothy due to heavy proteinuria. Edema involving the face, especially the periorbital region, arms, and genitalia. There may be ascites. There will not be high jugular pressure or pulmonary edema unless the renal or cardiac failure ispresent. There may be features of the underlying causes, such as a butterfly facial rash in systemic lupus erythematosus,

Treatment. ***A.* General measures**. Dietary sodium restriction and a thiazide diuretics eg. bendrofluazide 5 mg daily. If the patient is not responding, then they need frusemide 40-120 mgdaily with the addition of amiloride 5 mg daily, and the serum potassium should be monitored carefully. A normal protein is recommended as a high-protein intake confers no benefits. Infusionof albumin has only a transient effect and is only used in diuretic-resistant patients **B Specific measures**. 1. Minimal change glomerular lesion. High-dose corticosteroids with prednisolone 60mg daily for 8 weeks may correct the urinary protein leak in more than 95% of the children. Adults may need a few months of steroid therapy as the response rate is lower if remission lastsfor 4 years after the steroid therapy, then further relapse is uncommon. One-third of the patients relapse after steroid therapy, and in these patients, the remission is induced with steroid therapy again, and a course of cyclophosphamide 3 mg/kg daily is given for 6-8 weeks. 2. Membranous glomerulonephritis. There is controversy as to the value of steroids and immunosuppressive therapy, as many patients do well without any specific treatment 3. Other causes. Remission occurs if the underlying disease is treated. For patients with systemic lupus erythematosus, treatment with steroids and cyclophosphamide may induce long-term remission. Prolonged anticoagulation is required in a patient with renal vein thrombosis. Early detection of infection andaggressive infection treatment with antibiotics, as sepsis is a main cause of death in nephrotic patients. Acute tubular necrosis may develop as renal ischemia occurs due to low blood volume and septicemia. Thus, albumin infusion combined with mannitol may initiate a diuresis in oliguric renal failure.

Question 210 Differentiate orthostatic proteinuria (orthostatic albuminuria) and latent glomerulonephritis.

Orthostatic proteinuria. This is considered a benign condition where proteinuria is not detectedafter a period of hours lying flat, especially on rising in the morning, and subsequent urine specimen show proteinuria.

Latent glomerulonephritis. This is the sign of glomerular inflammation indicating the exacerbation of a pre-axis glomerular disease, such as IgA nephropathy where proteinuria ispresent and is not orthostatic dependent.

Question 211 Outline the prophylaxis measures for the recurrence of urolithiasis.

Prophylaxis measures for the recurrence of urolithiasis. A. Idiopathic stone-formers where no metabolic abnormality is present. The mainstay of prevention is the maintenance of a high intake offluid throughout the night and ensuring a urine output of 2-2.5 liters per day. B. Idiopathic hypercalciuria. Dietary calcium restriction is recommended, and to avoid vitamin D supplements. Al fluid intake is recommended, and the advice of a dietitian is helpful. If hypercalciuria persists and stone formation continues, a thiazide e.g., benzo thiazides 2.5-5 mg each morning is used. Thiazides reduce urinary calcium excretion with a direct effect on the renal tubule. C. Mixed infective stones. It can be prevented by high fluid intake and control of bacteria with antibacterialagents. D. Uric acid stones. It may be prevented by long-term use of a xanthine oxidase inhibitor, allopurinol, to maintain the serum urate and urinary uric acid excretion in the normal range. A high fluid intake is also recommended. E. Cystine stones. This can be prevented and will dissolve slowly if a high fluid intake of 5 liters of what must be drunk daily. Many patients cannot tolerate this regimen. Thus, a long-term chelating agent, penicillamine, may convert the cystine stone to a more soluble penicillamine-cysteine complex. E. Hyperoxaluria with calcium oxalate stones. A high fluid intake and dietary oxalate restriction are recommended.

Question 212 Discuss the milk-alkali syndrome

Milk-alkaline syndrome. It is due to excessive ingestion of calcium and absorbable antacids, such as milk or calcium carbonate. This syndrome can present as acute, subacute, and chronic, andall have hypercalcemia, alkalosis, and renal failure. The ingestion of hypercalcemia after meals would lead to increased bicarbonate resorption, which then leads to alkalosis. There would also be increased sodium excretion and some depletion of total-body water. The alkalosis would again cause enhancement of calcium resorption in the distal nephron, thus aggravating hypercalcemia. This cycle continues if the calcium and the absorbable alkaliare ingested. Acute milk-alkali syndrome is presented as weakness, myalgia, irritability, and apathy. If the intake of calcium and alkali is stopped, the renal function's impairment will reverse rapidly. Subacute milk-alkali syndrome is when renal failure is reversible over a period of weeks after withdrawal of excessive calcium and alkali ingestion. The chronic and long-standing milk-alkali syndrome is due to long-term ingestion of calcium and alkali and is presented with severe hypercalcemia, irreversible renal failure, and phosphate retention, which may be accompanied by ectopic calcification. Dialysis is important in this instance to prevent death.

Question 213 Differentiate urinary frequency and polyuria.

Urinary frequency. It is the passage of small urine volumes commonly seen in urinarytract infections.

Polyuria. It is a persistent, large increase in urine output, usually associated with nocturia. It canbe due to excessive intake of water, increased excretion of solute, as in hyperglycemia and glycosuria, or a defective renal concentrating ability or failure to produce anti-diuretic hormone.

Question 214 Discuss the clinical manifestations associated with diseases of the blood.

Clinical manifestations associated with diseases of the blood.

The patient may present with non-specific symptoms, such as fatigue, headaches, and faintness which can be normal in the general population. The others include breathlessness, angina on effort, intermittent claudication, and palpitation. The patient may present with non-specific signs, such as pallor, tachycardia, systolic flow murmur, cardiac failure, and maybe papilledema, and retinal hemorrhages after an acute bleed. Specific signs of different types of diseases of the blood include, Koilonychia - spoon-shaped nails seen in iron deficiency anemia, Jaundice - found in hemolytic anemia, Bone deformities - found in thalassemia major, Leg ulcers - occur in sickle-cell disease, Bleeding gums, and epitaxies -

in aplastic anemia, Splenomegaly with anemia and leg ulcers - occurs in hereditary spherocytosis, Acute drug-induced hemolysis - occurs in glucose-6-phosphate dehydrogenase deficiency. Severe itching after a hot bath occurs in polycythemia vera, Splenomegaly with lethargy and weight loss, and in myelofibrosis, Easy bruising, epistaxis platelets disorders, Hemarthroses with a joint deformity - occurs in coagulation disorders. Deep vein thrombosis, pulmonary thrombosis - occurs in thrombotic disorders.

Question 215 Give classification of the anemias

Classification of the anemias the classification is based on the mean corpuscular volume (MCV)
A. Low MVC or microcytes 1. Iron deficiency 2. Thalassemia 3. Anemia of chronic disease 4. Sideroblastic anemia B. High MVC or macrocytes 1. Megaloblastic anemia – Vitamin B12 or folate deficiency 2. Normoblastic anemia – Liver disease, alcohol, hemolysis C. Normal MCV 1.Acute blood loss 2. Anemia of chronic disease 3. Infection 4. Collagen disease 5. Malignancy 6. Endocrine disease

Question 216 Discuss the characteristics of anemia due to iron deficiency.

Characteristics of anemia due to iron deficiency. The patient may present fatigue, headaches, faintness, breathlessness, angina on effort, intermittent claudication, and palpitations.The signs of tissue iron deficiency are mainly epithelial changes induced by the effect of inadequate iron in the cells, such as brittle nails, spoon-shaped nails, atrophy of the papillae of the tongue, angular stomatitis, brittle hair and a syndrome of dysphagia and glossitis (Plummer-Vinson syndrome)

Question 217Outline specific therapy for pernicious anemia (addisonism).

Specific therapy for pernicious anemia. It is treated with intramuscular injection of hydroxocobalamin 1000 microgram to a total of 5000-6000 micrograms over the course of 3 weeks. Then 1000 micrograms are necessary every 3 months for the rest of the patient's life. Clinical improvement may occur within 48 hours, and reticulocytotic may be seen 2-3 days afterstarting therapy. The peripheral neuropathy improvement may occur over 6-12 months, but the long-standing spinal cord damage is irreversible. In some patients, the rapid regeneration of the blood may deplete the body's iron reserves, and recovery is halted. To prevent this, ferrous sulfate 200 mg daily should be given together with the therapy.

Question 218 What is the significance of exercise-march hemoglobinuria?

Significance of exercise-march hemoglobinuria. Damage to the red cells in the feet is associated with prolonged marching and results in mechanical hemolytic anemia. The red cellsare injured by physical trauma in the circulation and may cause cell lysis or may be followed by resealing of the red cell membrane with the formation of distorted red cells or fragments, which may circulate for a while before being destroyed prematurely in the reticuloendothelial system.

Question 219 Mention five types of megaloblastic anemia other than pernicious anemia.

Five types of megaloblastic anemia. 1. Vitamin B12 deficiency or abnormal vitamin B12 metabolism with normal intrinsic factors. 2. Folic acid deficiency or abnormal folate metabolism. 3. Congenital enzyme deficiencies in DNA synthesis, such as orotic aciduria. 4.Therapy with drugs interfering with DNA synthesis. 5. Myelodysplasia.

Question 220 Describe and give treatment for the most important complication of hemophilia.

The most important complication of hemophilia is hemarthroses which are common and may lead tojoint deformity and crippling if adequate treatment is not given.

Treatment. Bleeding is controlled by intravenous administration of high-purity factor VIII concentrate. The factor VIII level should be raised to 20-30% of normal, and the level should be raised to 50% for severe bleeding. There may be antibodies to factor VIII: C. Management of such patients is difficult. Patients can be given extremely high doses of factor VIIT, recombinant factor VIIa, purified factor V111, or factor IX concentrates containing activated factor X.

Question 221 Give the differential diagnosis in agranulocytosis (agranulocytosis angina)

Differential diagnosis in agranulocytosis. 1. Congenital - e.g., Kostmann's syndrome. 2. Racial -commoner in black races. 3. Viral infection 4. Severe bacterial infection - e.g., typhoid 5. Felty'ssyndrome 6. Autoimmune neutropenia 7. Pancytopenia - e.g., drug-induced marrow aplasia - clozapine, thiourea.

Question 222 Discuss the treatment of leukemia.

Treatment of leukemia. Acute leukemia. The aim of treatment is to destroy the leukemic clone ofcells without destroying the residual normal stem cell compartment where the hemopoietic tissues will be reputed.

Specific therapy. A Remission induction. The bulk of the tumor is destroyed by combination chemotherapy. The drugs used for acute lymphoblastic leukemia (ALL) are vincristine, L- asparaginase, daunorubicin, and methotrexate. And the drugs for acute myeloid leukemia (AML) aredaunorubicin, cytosine arabinoside, etoposide, and thioguanine. B. Remission consolidation. The residual disease is attacked by therapy during the consolidation phase. Drugs for ALL are daunorubicin, cytosine, and etoposide. And the drugs for AM are cytosine arabinoside, amacrine, and mitoxantrone. C. Remission maintenance. If the patient is in remission after the consolidation phasefor ALL, then a period of maintenance therapy is given consisting of a repeating cycle of drug administration for up to 2 years. The drugs given are vincristine, mercaptopurine, methotrexate.

Supportive therapy. A. Anemia - Treated with red cell concentrate infusion to maintain hemoglobin above 10 grams%. B. Bleeding - Treated with platelet transfusions. C Infection - Parenteral antibiotic therapy is essential for septicemia. Empirical therapy of gentamicin and azlocillin is given. Gram-positive infection may require vancomycin, especially for patients with an indwelling intravenous catheter. Oral and pharyngeal monilial infection is common, and prophylactic oral nystatin is given. Intravenous amphotericin is given for systemic fungal infection with candida or pulmonary aspergillosis. Herpes simplex infection around lips and nosemay require acyclovir prophylactically. D. Psychological support for the patients.

Allogeneic bone marrow transplantation (BMT). This is the only hope of a 'cure' for patients. Healthy marrow from a donor (histocompatibility siblings) is injected intravenously into a recipient who has obtained the conditioned ablation, which ablates the recipient's hemopoietic and immunological tissues. The injected cells will produce enough erythrocytes, granulocytes, and platelets in the marrow for the patient's needs in about 3-4 weeks, and it takesup to 3 years to regain good lymphocytic function and immunological stability.

Chronic leukemia.

A. Chronic myeloid leukemia No specific treatment is needed if the patient is asymptomatic, and the leukocyte count is not greatly elevated. Chemotherapy. Hydroxyurea is widely used to control the initial disease and improve the quality of life but cannot prolong life. Two types of treatment that can prolong life. 1. Alpha interferon can induce and maintain control ofthe disease in the chronic phase in about 70% of patients. 2. Allogeneic bone marrow transplant from a matched sibling donor provides the only means of obtaining long-term remission.

B. Myelofibrosis. Treatment is largely supportive of blood transfusion. Hydroxyurea can beused to reduce splenic size and for very high leukocyte count. Splenectomy for grossly enlarged spleen. Bone marrow transplantation should be considered for young patients.

C Chronic lymphocytic leukemia. 1. Patient with no anemia or thrombocytopenia and less than three areas of lymphoid enlargement - No specific treatment is required. Life expectancy is normal in older patients, and the patient should be assured. 2. Patient with no anemia or thrombocytopenia with three or more involved areas. - No treatment may be required if asymptomatic. Chemotherapy with chlorambucil may be started in symptomatic patients. Local radiotherapy to lymph nodes causes discomfort. 3.

Patients with anemia and thrombocytopenia, regardless of the number of lymphoid enlargements - Anemia should be treatedwith red cell transfusion. Bone marrow failure is treated with prednisolone.

D. Hairy cell leukemia. Alpha interferon is very effective in controlling the disease.E. Prolymphocytic leukemia. Leukapheresis, splenectomy, and chemotherapy may be tried, but treatmentis usually unsuccessful.

E Myelodysplastic syndrome. Supportive treatment with blood and platelet transfusion. Allogeneic transplantation may be tried for a younger patient, but the success rate is low.

Question 223 Give the treatment and common complication of polycythemia vera.

Treatment of polycythemia vera. The aim is to keep the packed cell volume below 45% and theplatelet below 400 000 and prevent disease complications. A Venesection. It relieves many symptoms of the disease. About 500 ml of blood is removed, if necessary, to be repeated after 1 or 2 days. B. Chemotherapy. Continuous or intermittent treatment with agents, such as busulphan or hydroxyurea, controls thrombocytosis. C. Radioactive 322. Itis used in elderly patients, and one dose may give control for up to 18 months. D. Allopurinol is given to block uric acid production. Avoid hot baths to lessen the pruritus.

Complications of polycythemia vera 1. Thromboses and hemorrhages. 2. Myelofibrosis. 3. Acutemyeloblastic leukemia.

Question 224 What does the term auto-immune hemolytic diseases refer to?

Auto-immune hemolytic diseases. This is a condition where antibodies are produced in one individual, which reacts with the red cells of another. This is seen in hemolytic disease of the newborn, hemolytic transfusion reactions. After allogeneic bone marrow, renal, liver, or cardiac transplantation when donor lymphocytes transferred in the allograft may produce red cellantibodies against the recipient and cause hemolytic anemia.

Question 225 Discuss the various causes of the hemorrhagic group of diseases.

Causes of the hemorrhagic group of diseases.

A. Vascular disorder. 1. Hereditary hemorrhagic telangiectasia - recurrent epitaxies and gastrointestinal bleeding are major problems. 2. Severe infections - Septicemia, meningococcal infections, typhoid. 3. Henoch-Schoenlein purpura. 4. Drugs - steroids, sulphonamides. 5. Others
- senile purpura, easy bruising syndrome, and scurvy.

B. Platelet disorder Bleeding due to thrombocytopenia or abnormal platelet function. Causes of thrombocytopenia - 1. Impaired production. a. Bone marrow failure - leukemia, aplastic anemia,megaloblastic anemia. b. Reduction in megakaryocytes - drugs like co-trimoxazole, viral infections. 2. Excessive destruction. a. Immune - Autoimmune thrombocytopenic purpura, post-transfusion purpura. b. Coagulation - Disseminated intravascular coagulation 3. Sequestration - Hypersplenism 4. Dilutional loss - Massive transfusion of stored blood.

C. Coagulation disorders. 1. Inherited coagulation disorders. a. Hemophilia A b. Hemophilia B c.Von Willebrand's disease. 2. Acquired coagulation disorders a. Vitamin K deficiency b. Liver disease - Reduced synthesis of coagulation factors, thrombocytopenia from hypersplenism inportal hypertension. c. Disseminated intravascular coagulation, d. Excessive fibrinolysis, e. Massive transfusion of stored blood has reduced levels of factors V and VIII.

Question 226 Define and give treatment for primary splenic neutropenia.

Primary splenic neutropenia It is the condition where neutropenia is due to an increased rate ofdestruction of neutrophils.

Treatment of the underlying causes like hematological disorders, portal hypertension, rheumatoid arthritis, and lymphoma. Splenectomy may be required for severe anemia or thrombocytopenia.

Question 227 What is the treatment for cirrhotic splenomegaly (Banti's syndrome)?

Treatment for cirrhotic splenomegaly (Banti's syndrome). Banti's syndrome is congestive splenomegaly with hypersplenism associated with cirrhosis and portal hypertension. Splenectomy is sometimes required for severe anemia due to hypersplenism or thrombocytopenia.

Question 228 List the conditions included in the diagnostic category of lymphosarcoma.

The conditions included in the diagnostic category of lymphosarcoma. 1. Small lymphocytic lymphoma 2. Follicular small-cleaved lymphoma 3. Follicular mixed histiocytic lymphoma 4. Follicular large-cell lymphoma 5. Diffuse small-cleaved lymphoma. 6. Diffuse mixed histiocyticlymphoma 7. Diffuse large-cell lymphoma 8. Immunoblastic lymphoma 9. Lymphoblastic lymphoma 10. Small non-cleaved lymphoma

Question 229 What findings are of diagnostic importance in multiple myeloma (plasmacytic myeloma).

Diagnostic importance in multiple myeloma. 1. Renal impairment - high urea, creatinine, and electrolyte levels. 2. Hypercalcemia. 3. Bone fractures - lytic lesions in the skull 4. Protein electrophoresis - monoclonal band. 5. Bone marrow failure - infiltration by plasma cells.

Question 230 What symptoms or findings suggest the diagnosis of sub-leukemic (aleukemic)leukemic?

Symptoms or findings suggest the diagnosis of sub-leukemic. 1. Cutaneous chloromas (granulocytic sarcomas). 2. Absences of blasts in the peripheral smear. 3. The total white countin the peripheral blood is not raised.

References

1. Harrison ‘s Principles of Internal Medicine – 13th Edition
2. Davidson ‘s Principles and Practices of Medicine – 17th Edition.

Question 231 Discuss the diagnosis and various forms of Hodgkin's disease.

Diagnosis and various forms of Hodgkin's disease. Diagnosis is based on clinical features andinvestigations.

Symptoms. 1. Painless lymph node enlargement, mainly the cervical lymph node.
2. The 'B' symptoms - are fever, night sweats, and weight loss of >10% of body weight. 3. Others - e.g., pruritus, fatigue, anorexia, and alcohol-induced pain at the site of enlarged lymph nodes. 4. Symptoms due to other organs - e.g., liver, bone, lung. Signs. 1. Peripheral lymph node enlargement 2. Enlargement of the spleen/liver depends on the stage. Investigations. 1. Erythrocyte sedimentation rate - raised. 2. Chest X-ray - mediastinal widening. 3. CT scan - enlargement of intrathoracic, abdominal, or pelvic lymph nodes. 4. Lymph node biopsy - Sternberg-Reed cells with lymphocytes and histiocytes.

<u>Various forms of Hodgkin's disease are based on staging.</u>

I. Involvement of a single lymph node region or a single extra lymphatic organ or site.

II. Involvement of two or more lymph node regions on the same side of the diaphragmor one or more lymph node regions plus an extra lymphatic site.

III. Involvement of lymph node regions on both sides of the diaphragm with or withoutsplenic enlargement.

IV. Involvement of one or more extra lymphatic organs, e.g., lung, liver, bone marrow, with or without lymph node involvement.

Question 232 In what conditions may rupture of the spleen occur?

<u>Conditions that may rupture the spleen.</u> 1. Direct or remote trauma. 2. Infectious diseases suchas Malaria, Typhoid fever, EB virus-induced infectious

mononucleosis

Question 233 Discuss the etiology of diabetes mellitus.

Etiology of diabetes mellitus. The discussion on etiology can be divided into insulin-dependent diabetes mellitus (IDDM), non-insulin-dependent diabetes mellitus (NIDDM), and secondarydiabetes.

Etiology of IDDM. A Genetic IDDM is not genetically predetermined, but an increased susceptibility to the disease may be inherited. B. Identical twins. They have a 30-35% chance ofdeveloping the disease. C. Inheritance. The child of an IDDM patient has an increased chance of developing IDDM. This risk is greater with a diabetic father (1 in 20-40) than a diabetic mother (1 in 40-80). If one child in a family has IDDM, each sibling has a 1 in 20 risks of developing diabetes. If the sibling is HLA-identical, the risk rises to 1 in 6. More than 90% of IDDM patients carry HLA-DR3 or DR4 compared with 40% of the general population. D. Autoimmunity. Presences of islet cell antibodies, insulin autoantibodies, insulitis, immunosuppression following diagnosis delays pancreatic beta-cell destruction and associationwith other organ-specific autoimmune diseases, such as pernicious anemia, and Addison's disease.

Etiology of NIDDM. A. Genetics. Identical twins of a patient with NIDDM have 90% concordance, and about 25% of other patients have a first-degree relative with NIDDM. B. Noevidence of immune disturbance and no HLA links.

Etiology of secondary diabetes. A. Liver disease - cirrhosis. B. Pancreatic disease - cystic fibrosis, chronic pancreatitis, hemochromatosis, carcinoma of the pancreas,

pancreatectomy. C. Endocrine diseases - Cushing's syndrome, acromegaly, thyrotoxicosis, pheochromocytoma, glucagonoma. D. Drug-induced diseases - thiazides diuretics, corticosteroids. E. Insulin-receptorabnormalities - congenital lipoatrophy, acanthosis nigricans. F. genetic syndrome e.g.
Friedreich 's ataxia, myotonic dystrophy.

Question 234 List the complications which may occur in an inadequately controlled diabetic.

Complications that occur in an inadequately controlled diabetic. Acute complications. 1. Hypoglycemia. 2. Diabetic ketoacidosis. 3. Non-kenotic hyperosmolar diabetic coma. 4. Lacticacidosis - in association with biguanide therapy. B. Long-term complications. 1. Diabetic retinopathy. 2. Diabetic neuropathy - polyneuropathy, mononeuropathy, and autonomic neuropathy. 3. Diabetic foot - neuropathic and ischemic foot. 4. Diabetic nephropathy.

Question 235 What factors play an important role in the development and prognosis of acidosis and coma?

Factors that play an important role in the development of acidosis and coma. 1. Previouslyundiagnosed diabetes. 2. Interruption of insulin therapy. 3. Stress of intercurrent illness. 4. Consumption of glucose-rich fluids 5. Concurrent medication, such as thiazide diuretics or steroids.

Factors that play important in the prognosis of acidosis and coma. 1. Advanced age of thepatient - poor prognosis. 2. Frequency of intercurrent illness.

Question 236 What are the indications for insulin therapy?

Indications for insulin therapy. 1. Insulin-dependent diabetes mellitus. 2. Non-insulin dependentdiabetes mellitus. 3. Diabetic ketoacidosis. 4. Non-ketotic hyperosmolar diabetic coma. 5. Hyperkalemia.

Question 237 How would you diagnose a case of diabetes mellitus?

Diagnosis of diabetes mellitus. 1. In the symptomatic patient, single elevated blood glucose indicates diabetes 2. In asymptomatic or mildly symptomatic patients, the diagnosis is made c a.Fasting venous blood glucose levels above 6.7 mmol/liter. b. Random values above 10 mmol/liter in whole venous blood. 3. In true borderline cases, an oral glucose tolerance test can be used. The blood glucose over 6.7 mmol/liter or when the 2-hour value is over 10 mmindicates diabetes.

Question 238 Outline the treatment of diabetic coma.

Treatment of diabetic coma A. Replacement of fluid loss. Normal saline 0.9% is given, 1 liter in 30 minutes, then 1 liter in 1 hour, the 2 hours, then 1 liter in 4 hours, and 1 liter in 6 hours. Add KCI 20 mmol in B. Replacement of deficient insulin. Insulin intravenous 6-unit stat, then 6-unit hourly by infusion. C. Replacement of electrolyte losses. Potassium levels must be monitored 2 hourlies for the first 8 hours to avoid 1 complication of hypokalemia and hyperkalemia. D. Monitoring of the blood glucose - hourly monitoring initially for 8 hours. E. Restoring the acid-base balance. Isotonic 1.26% bicarbonate solution if pH is below 7.0. Bicarbonate replaces necessary if the patient's renal function is healthy and can compensate for the metabolic acidosis. E. Replacement of energy losses. Give infusion of 5% dextrose solution with 20 mmol/liter of KCl to replace infusion when the plasma glucose falls to near-normal values. G. seek the underlying causes by investigation, such as chest X-ray, urine, and blood cultures. Treat infection aggressively with broad-spectrum antibiotics. H. bladder cathectic if no urine output in 2 hours, nasogastric tube to prevent aspiration, subcutaneous heparin in comatose patients, central venousline in comatose patients.

Question 239 Describe the prognosis of nondiabetic acidosis.

Prognosis of nondiabetic acidosis. It can lead to the simulation of the respiratory center and cause Kussmaul's sign or air hunger. Acidosis is negatively inotropic and thus causes cardiac depression. Severe acidosis cause vasoconstriction, resulting in the redistribution of blood from the peripheriesto the central circulation and increasing the systemic venous pressure, which may worsen pulmonary edema caused by cardiac depression. Acidosis can cause arteriolar vasodilatation leading to hypotension. Severe acidosis can lead to confusion and fits. Acidosis can also stimulate potassium loss from cells leading to hypokalemia.

Question 240 Give the usual causes, clinical picture, and treatment of hypoglycemia in a patientreceiving insulin.

Cause of hypoglycemia. 1. Missed, delayed, or inadequate meal. 2. Unusual or unexpected exercise. 3. Alcohol. 4. Poorly designed insulin regime. 5. Sepsis. 6. Excessive insulin 7. Others -severe liver disease, adrenal insufficiency, salicylate poisoning

Clinical picture. Symptoms. 1. Autonomic - sweating, trembling, pounding heart, hunger, anxiety. 2. Neuroglycopenic - confusion, drowsiness, unable to concentrate, in coordination. 3. Others - nausea, tiredness, headache. Signs. Moist skin and tongue, full pulse, shallow breathing,brisk reflexes.

Treatment. 1. If the patient is drowsy, fitting, or has a very low blood glucose level, Give 50 ml of 50% dextrose intravenous or glucagon 1 mg intravenous, intramuscular, or subcutaneous Recheck blood glucose after 5 minutes and again after 30 minutes. 2. If hypoglycemia recurs or is likely to recur - Start 10% dextrose 1 liter 12 hourly intravenous. Adjust the rate to keep the blood glucoselevel at 5-10 mmol/liter. 3. Reassess the insulin regime for patient compliance and its design.

Question 241 Give the differential diagnosis of insulinoma.

Differential diagnosis of insulinoma. 1. Psychiatric disorders, such as pseudodementia in elderly patients. 2. Epilepsy. 3. Cardiovascular disease. 4. Advanced neoplasia and cachexia causing hypoglycemia. 5. Tumors, such as sarcoma, may secrete insulin-like growth factor 1, causinghypoglycemia.

Question 242 What is the significance of the diseases of inborn errors of metabolism?

Significance of the disease of inborn errors of metabolism. The genetic etiology of many inborn errors of metabolism has been identified with the abnormalities of the structure or function of DNA and the pattern of their inheritance mapped by the study of the biochemical disorder. The vast majority of the inborn errors of metabolism are rare, some with good prognosis, and some are fatal in their outcome. Recognition of the diseases of the inborn errors of metabolism has helped prevent further damage, e.g., a diet low in phenylalanine in phenylketonuria is tefirst months of life will prevent brain damage. There is inborn carbohydrate, amino acid metabolism errors, Lysosomal storage diseases, cystinosis, amyloidosis, and porphyria.

Question 243 Outline the treatment of gout.

Treatment of gout.

Acute attacks. Acute gout is treated with anti-inflammatory drugs. 1. Indomethacin 50 mg threeto four times daily should provide relief within 24-48 hours. Then the dose can be reduced to 25mg three to four times a day. Azapropazone 600 mg twice daily is the other alternative. 2.
Intramuscular adrenocorticotropin (ACTH) is very effective in difficult cases. 3. Effusion in large joints should be aspirated, and a corticosteroid injected to reduce inflammation

Long-term therapy. Measures to reduce the uric acids once the acute attack is settled.

1. Weight reduction 2. Reduction in alcohol intake. 3. Avoid food and drinks containing high levels of purine, e.g., beers and beans. 4. Good fluid intake S. Withdrawal of drugs like salicylatesand thiazides. 6. Allopurinol is the drug of choice, 300 mg daily and 100 mg in renal

disease. Allopurinol should be started only after 4 weeks from the last acute attack as it may precipitatean acute attack itself. Probenecid is an alternative in patients who are allergic to allopurinol.

Question 244 What is the cause of obesity?

Causes of obesity. 1. Simple obesity - intake of calories must exceed expenditure. 2. Hormonalimbalance in women, e.g., postmenopausal or when taking contraceptive pills. 3. Genetic syndromes - Prader-Willi syndrome, Laurence-Moon-Biedl syndrome. 4. Hypothyroidism. 5. Cushing's syndrome. 6. Stein-Leventhal syndrome. 7. Drug-induced - e.g., corticosteroids. 8. Hypothalamic damages - e.g., due to trauma or tumor.

Question 245 Discuss the treatment of atherosclerosis.

Treatment of atherosclerosis. The patients should have their serum cholesterol determined by their pimayphysicians. Discontinuance of smoking and dietary management and pharmacological management when the serum cholesterol is above 200 mg/dL are certain measures to prevent morbidity from atherosclerosis.

Atherosclerotic occlusion of the aorta and its branches are a common cause of disability, An Occlusive atherosclerosis of the aorta and iliac arteries. 1. Patient may receive pentoxifylline 400mg three times daily for claudication pain and beta-blockers for angina. 2. Arterial prosthesis bypass for complex aortoiliac occlusive disease. 3. Thromboendarterectomy for occlusion in the common iliac arteries 4. Endovascular surgical techniques, such as percutaneous transluminal angioplasty. Atherectomy and laser may be used.

B. Atherosclerotic occlusive disease of the femoral and popliteal arteries. 1. Arterial graft - using theautogenous vein graft of the great saphenous vein to bypass the occluded segments. 2. Thromboendarterectomy with the removal of the central occluding core if the occlusion is short. 3. Endovascular Surgery - balloon angioplasty to forcefully dilate the narrow areas or mechanical atherectomy to remove the atheroma from the lumen of the artery or using laser or thermal angioplasty to vaporize the occlusive material.

C Atherosclerotic occlusion of the coronary arteries. 1 Percutaneous transluminal coronary angioplasty (PTCA) The aim is dilation which ruptures the atheromatous plaque with some resorption of the intraluminal debris. Coronary stenoses can be dilated by the inflation of a balloon under high pressure. It can be used in multivessel disease with multiple lesions. 2. Coronary artery bypass grafting (CABG). Grafts from the internal mammary arteries or the saphenous veincan be used for CABG. One to five anastomoses can be performed between the aorta and the coronary arteries distal to the obstruction. 3. Revascularization procedures. Use catheter devices to remove atheromatous material (atherectomy) and laser catheters. Intracoronary stents can maintain vessel patency in patients with acute closure during PTCA or with restenosis.

Question 246 Give the diagnosis of secondary amyloidosis.

Diagnosis of secondary amyloidosis. 1. Microscopic examination of biopsy, such as gingival, renal, rectal, or surgical specimens, is diagnostic. 2. Amyloid binds

Congo red dye in tissues and emits apple green fluorescence with ultraviolet light. 3. Fine-needle biopsy of the subcutaneousabdominal fat is a simple and reliable test to diagnose secondary amyloidosis.

Question 247 Discuss the etiology of osteoporosis.

Etiology of osteoporosis. There are two types of osteoporosis. Type 1 is the typical postmenopausal osteoporosis which is due to estrogen deficiency. Type 2 is senile osteoporosis due to senile secondary hyperparathyroidism leading to cortical bone resorption: There are some factors which are important for the pathogenesis of type 2 osteoporosis. They are: 1. Less sunshine. 2. Lower calcium intake 3. Less vitamin D-containing foods 4. Less vitamin D synthesis in the skin.

There are risk factors for the etiology of osteoporosis which are:

Endogenous

1. Female

2. Asian or Caucasian 3. Small stature

4. Thin physique 5. Family history

6. Nulliparity. 7. Early menopause

8. Advanced age

Exogenous 1. Reduced physical exercise. 2. Cigarette smoking. 3. Alcohol abuse. 4. Aluminum antacids. 5. Surgical menopause. 6. Steroid therapy.

Diseases 1. Endocrine - Cushing's syndrome, diabetes mellitus, thyrotoxicosis, hypogonadism, acromegaly. 2. Rheumatoid arthritis. 3. Chronic renal failure.

Question 248 Mention the common diseases of the pituitary gland.

Common diseases of the pituitary gland. 1. Isolated deficiency of pituitary hormones, e.g.,Kallman's syndrome. 2. Pituitary apoplexy. 3. Sheehan's syndrome. 4. Pituitary tumors - prolactinoma, craniopharyngiomas, Cushing's disease, acromegaly.

Question 249 Outline the clinical manifestations and findings of panhypopituitarism (Simmonds's disease).

Clinical manifestations and findings of panhypopituitarism (Simonds 's disease). The signs and symptoms depend upon the extent of hypothalamic and pituitary deficiencies. Loss of libido, amenorrhea, and impotence are symptoms of gonadotrophin. Thus, gonadal deficiencies, while hyperprolactinemia may cause galactorrhea and hypogonadism. GH deficiency is clinically 'silent' except in children. Secondary hypothyroidism and adrenal failure lead to tiredness, slowness of thought and action, and mild hypotension. Long-standing panhypopituitarism may give the classical picture of pallor with hairlessness. Some important syndromes related to hypopituitarism: 1. Kallman's syndrome - isolated gonadotrophin deficiency, which leads to hypogonadism. 2. Sheahan 's syndrome - pituitary infarction following postpartum hemorrhage. 3. Pituitary apoplexy - a pituitary tumor may cause an infarct or hemorrhage into itself. 4. Empty Sellasyndrome - defect in the diaphragm and extension of the subarachnoid space (cisternal herniation) or may follow spontaneous infarction of a tumor.

Question 250 Discuss the diagnosis of hyperthyroidism.

Diagnosis of hyperthyroidism. Diagnosis can be obtained from the clinical presentation and investigations of hyperthyroidism. Clinical presentation. Symptoms. Increased appetite, restlessness, tremors, palpitation, heat intolerance, diarrhea, eye complaints, oligomenorrhea. Signs. Hyperkinesis, exophthalmos, goiter with bruit, tachycardia and atrial fibrillation, warm vasodilated peripheries, proximal myopathy, pretibial myxedema. The eye signs, pretibial myxedema, and thyroid acropachy occur only in Graves' disease. In the elderly, atrial fibrillationis frequent, with other tachycardias and heart failure. Children are presented with excessive heightor excessive growth rate or with behavior problems like hyperactivity. Investigations. Serum TSH is depressed with a raised serum 13 and T4. Microsomal antibodies and thyroglobulin antibodies are present in most cases of Graves' disease.

Question 251 Outline the treatment of hypothyroidism.

Treatment of hypothyroidism. Replacement therapy with T4 is given for life. In the young and fit, 100 micrograms daily are given, and 50 micrograms daily for the old and frail. Patients with ischemic heart disease require lower doses, especially if the hypothyroidism is severe and long-standing. The patient should be given 25 micrograms daily and perform serial EKG, increasing the dose at 2-6-week intervals if angina does not occur or worsen and the EKG does not deteriorate. If progress is satisfactory, T4 100 microgram daily is given. Adequacy of a replacement should be assessed clinically and by thyroid function tests after 6 weeks on a steady dose to restore the TSH to the normal range. If serum TSH remains high, the doseof T4 should be increased in 25 microgram increments, and the tests repeated 6 weeks later,

The usual maintenance dose is 100-200 micrograms given as a single daily dose. Clinical improvement on T4 may not begin for 2 weeks, and full resolution of symptoms may take 6months. The importance of life-long therapy must be emphasized to the patient.

Question 251 Give a clinical picture of acute thyroiditis.

The clinical picture of thyroiditis. It is seen commonly in females aged 20-40. This form of hyperthyroidism is characterized by pain in the region of the thyroid gland, which radiates to theangle of the jaw and the ears and is made worse by swallowing, coughing, and movement of the neck. The thyroid is usually palpably enlarged and tender. Systemic upset is common.

Question 252 Discuss the relationship of the thymus gland to myasthenia gravis.

Relationship of the thymus gland to myasthenia gravis.

Thymic hyperplasia is found in 70% of myasthenic patients below the age of 40 years. In 10% ofpatients, a thymic tumor is found, and antibodies to striated muscle can be demonstrated in these patients. Young patients without thymoma have an increased association with HLA-B8 and DR3.

Question 253 List the causes, clinical findings, and treatment of hyperparathyroidism.

Causes of hyperthyroidism. A. Primary hyperparathyroidism. 1. Single adenoma 2. Multiple adenomata 3. Nodular hyperplasia. 4. Parathyroid carcinoma. B. Secondary hyperparathyroidism. 1. Chronic renal failure. 2. Malabsorption. 3. Osteomalacia and rickets C.Tertiary hyperparathyroidism - due to autonomous parathyroid hyperplasia after long-standing secondary hyperparathyroidism, most often in renal failure.

Clinical findings. The patient will present with malaise, nausea, vomiting, constipation, and weight loss. Later, there may be weakness, drowsiness, poor concentration, memory loss, and depression,

There may be renal colic from stones, polyuria/nocturia, hematuria, and hypertension. There maybe bone pain and abdominal pain. Primary hyperparathyroidism may present as local swelling of the mandible, due to the cyst. Deposition of calcium pyrophosphate crystal within articular cartilage and affects the menisci at the knees and can result in secondary degenerativearthritis. Corneal calcification, ectopic calcification in the arterial walls and soft tissues of hands,peptic ulceration, myopathy, and pruritus.

Treatment. For asymptomatic patients over 65 years with serum calcium levels less than 3.0 mmol/L, no treatment is necessary except for review every 6-12 months. The treatment for primary hyperparathyroidism is the surgical removal of the adenoma, and for the hyperplasia, all 4 glands are removed, and some of the excised tissue is transplanted in the forearm. Patients withhypercalcemic crises where the serum calcium is more than 3.5 mmol/L. This is a medical emergency, and the aim is fluid replacement, correcting the electrolyte imbalance, and lowering serum calcium levels. Fluids intravenously 3-4 liters daily of saline for 2-3 days. Intravenous diphosphates e.g., etidronate disodium, sodium clodronate, and pamidronate disodium, for hypercalcemia of malignancy. The intravenous dose of etidronate is 7.5 mg/kg daily for 3 days. Prednisolone 30-60 mg daily is effective, especially in myeloma, sarcoidosis, and vitamin D excess. Treatment of secondary hyperparathyroidism depends on the primary pathology, and sometimes, steroids may be useful.

Question 254 What symptoms and findings are suggestive of pheochromocytoma?

Symptoms and findings of pheochromocytoma. The patient may present with anxiety or panicattacks, palpitation, tremors, sweating, headaches, flushing, nausea, vomiting, weight loss, constipation or diarrhea, Raynaud's phenomenon, chest pain, and polyuria or nocturia. Some common findings are hypertension which may be intermittent or constant, tachycardia or arrhythmias, bradycardia, orthostatic hypotension, pallor or flushing, glycosuria, and fever.

Question 255 List the symptoms and signs of chronic adrenal insufficiency (Addison's disease).

Symptoms and signs of chronic adrenal insufficiency (Addison's disease) The patient may present with symptoms of weight loss, anorexia, malaise, weakness, fever, depression, impotenceor amenorrhea, nausea or vomiting, diarrhea, confusion, syncope from hypotension, abdominal pain, constipation, myalgia, joint or back pain, The common signs are buccal pigmentation, postural hypotension, pigmentation of new scars, general wasting, dehydration, loss of body hair and vitiligo.

Question 256 What is eunuchism?

Eunuchism is the deficiency of the testes or their secretion with impaired or decreased libidoand eunuchoid symptoms.

Question 257 Discuss and give the treatment of cryptorchidism (undescended testes).

Treatment of cryptorchidism (undescended testes). Medically, the patient should be tried with a course of chorionic gonadotrophin at about 6 years of age, or GnRH can be given intranasally for1-4 weeks. The success rate is about 40%. If the medical treatment is unsuccessful, then the testesshould be placed in the scrotum surgically. In the male descent of the testis, it may take an abnormal route and is liable to develop into a malignancy. Such testis in children should be surgically placed in the scrotum, or if discovered in adults, then it should be removed surgically or through orchidectomy as it may develop into a malignancy.

References

1. Harrison 's Principles of Internal Medicine – 13th Edition
2. Davidson 's Principles and Practices of Medicine – 17th Edition.

Question 258 Define primary aldosteronism.

Primary aldosteronism. Adrenal adenomas and bilateral adrenal hyperplasia can cause excessive production of aldosterone, leading to sodium retention and potassium loss and resulting in hypokalemia and hypertension with a clinical presentation like weakness, tetany nocturia and renaland retinal damage due to severe hypertension.

Question 259 Give the etiology of Loffler's syndrome (allergic pneumonia).

Etiology of Loffler's syndrome (allergic pneumonia). It is endomyocardial fibrosis in whichthere is severe fibrosis of the endocardium with eosinophilia resulting in restrictive cardiomyopathy.

Question 260 What effects do large amounts of androgen procedures have in females?

Effects of large amounts of androgen procedure in females. The female patients may develop deepening of the voice, frontotemporal balding, facial, axillary, and limb hairs, greasy skin, acne, marked obesity, oligomenorrhea or amenorrhea, and clitoromegaly.

Question 261 Discuss the etiology of gynecomastia.

Etiology of gynecomastia. A. Physiological 1. Neonatal. 2. Pubertal - occurs in about 50% of normal males and usually resolves spontaneously within 6-18 months or may need surgical removal after this duration, 3. Old age - full assessment is needed to exclude serious underlying diseases, such as bronchial carcinoma and testicular tumor. B. Hyperthyroidism. C. Liver disease. D. Estrogen-producing tumors from testis and adrenal. E. HCG-producing tumors from testis and lung, E Carcinoma of the breast. G. Starvation followed by refeeding. H. Drugs. 1. Estrogenic - estrogens, digitalis, cannabis, diamorphine. 2. Antiandrogens - spironolactone, cimetidine, cyproterone, 3. Others - gonadotrophins, cytotoxic.

Question 262 Explain the increase in free

estrogen content in the urine of patients with hepaticdisease.

Increase of free estrogen content in the urine of a patient with hepatic disease. In a person with normal hepatic function, the estrogens are converted in the liver to estriol and estrone and then conjugated with glucuronic acid or sulfate. Thus, any abnormalities in the hepatic catabolism ofestrogen due to hepatic disease will result in excessive estrogen in the body and are excreted as free estrogen in the urine.

Question 263 Discuss endocrine allergy.

Endocrine allergy endocrine allergy is the type II immunological response to the allergy due to endocrinal diseases. The autoimmune reactions occur in related groups reflecting the spectrumof autoimmune diseases ranging from the organ-specific to the non-organ-specific. A good example of a Type II antibody-mediated immunological response is the number of autoantibodiesformed to different thyroid antigens in autoimmune thyroid disease. The patients with one of the diseases in the organ-specific group tend to have an increased prevalence of autoantibodies in the target organs of other diseases. Some important autoimmune endocrinal diseases are Hashimoto's thyroiditis, primary myxedema, thyrotoxicosis, pernicious anemia, autoimmuneatrophic gastritis, autoimmune Addison's disease, Type 1 diabetes mellitus, myasthenia gravis, primary biliary cirrhosis, and chronic active hepatitis.

Question 264 Differentiate between arthritis and rheumatism.

Arthritis. It is the inflammation of the joint marked by pain, heat, redness, and swelling.

Rheumatism. A term used to represent any of a variety of disorders marked by inflammation, degeneration, or metabolic derangements of the connective tissue structures, especially the jointsand related structures, and clinically with pain, stiffness, and limitation of motions.

Question 265 Give the fundamentals concerned with the management of arthritis.

Fundamentals concerned with the management of arthritis.

1. Relief of the symptoms of arthritis
2. Suppression of active and progressive disease of arthritis.
3. Conservation and restoration of function in the affected joints. All these can be managed bytreatment of the patients with drugs, rest, physiotherapy, surgery, and modification of the environment with aids, appliances, housing, and occupation benefits.

Question 266 Give the differential diagnosis of rheumatoid arthritis (atrophic or chronic proliferative arthritis, arthritis deformans).

Differential diagnosis of rheumatoid arthritis. 1. Inflammatory joint diseases. Ankylosing spondylitis, Reiter's disease, psoriatic arthritis, juvenile chronic arthritis, Bechet's syndrome. 2. Infectious arthritis. Bacterial, viral and fungal 3. Connective tissue diseases. Systemic lupus erythematosus, progressive systemic sclerosis, polymyositis. 4. Crystal deposition diseases. Goutand chondrocalcinosis. 5. Osteoarthrosis. 6. Soft tissue pain. Epicondylitis, olecranon bursitis, trigger finger,

Dupuytren's contracture.

Question 267 Give the clinical manifestations and treatment of Reiter's syndrome.

Clinical manifestations of Reiter's syndrome. The patient is commonly a young male who presents with arthritis which begins within 2 weeks of enteric or venereal infection. The knees, ankles, and feet are the commonest sites of arthritis. The wrists and the other joints in the upper limb may be involved, and occasionally, there may be localized pain and tenderness in the spinedue to sacroiliitis. The arthritis is very acute initially and would resolve over the course of a few months. There would be urethritis which is associated with sterile urethral discharge, and mild dysuria. Circinate balanitis with a circle of erythema with a pale lesion on the penis is uncommon. There may be conjunctivitis which is mild and bilateral. Acute anterior uveitis maydevelop in some patients. There may be keratoderma blennorrhagica in patients with post-venereal Reiter's syndrome. It is characterized by intense scaling of the skin of the soles of the feet. Patients may present with a low-grade fever. Very rarely, there may be complications like pericarditis, aortitis, pleurisy, and peripheral neuropathy.

Treatment. Patients can be given non-steroidal anti-inflammatory agents, such as indomethacin. Itmay be necessary to aspirate an acutely inflamed joint and to inject the joints with a corticosteroid preparation in acute arthritis, which fails to respond quickly, and in chronic cases,sulphasalazine or azathioprine can be used.

Question 268 Outline the treatment of rheumatoid.

Treatment of rheumatoid.

Step 1. Assessment of the patient is part of the diagnostic process, and proper explanation, information, and reassurance must be provided for the patient as it affects the patient's lifestyle. The patient must be advised on weight reduction and control. A simple exercise to maintain joint mobility and muscle power. Plans must be made for the continuing care of the patient.

Step 2. Relief of symptoms with medications and other measures is the treatment's mainstay. Non-steroidal anti-inflammatory agents are more effective than simple analgesics. Drugs with minimal side effects should be tried for 1 week, such as piroxicam 20 mg daily. Therelief of night pain and morning stiffness is important, and this may be achieved with the slow-release indomethacin 75 mg at bedtime. Corticosteroids may be used in explosive rheumatoid arthritis in the elderly, such as 10 mg prednisolone daily. Rest in the hospital may be useful, and localized rest for the joints with splints. Intra-articular corticosteroid injections can be used fortroublesome joints to avoid the risk of systemic steroids.

Step 3. Long-term suppressive drug therapy with drugs like penicillamine, azathioprine, and methotrexate are used for progressive disease, troublesome extra-articular problems, failure of NSAIDS to control symptoms, and if excessive corticosteroids are used. Complete remission orvery effective disease suppression can be achieved, delaying or preventing joint destruction.

Step 4. Regular supervision is required to assess the disease's course and treat complications. Patients with articular complications with joints that have become stiff and painful require intra-articular injections of corticosteroids and exercises to mobilize the joint and improve muscle power. Deformities can also be corrected by steroid injections and exercise. Rupture of the knee joint is treated with aspiration, injection of corticosteroids, and rest.Painful feet may be treated with insoles. Replacement surgery for wrecked joints is possible and necessary. Replacement of the hip, knees, shoulders, elbows and small joints of the hands is possible. Excision arthroplasty is also of value. Patients who develop carpal tunnel syndrome may need an injection of corticosteroids or surgical decompression of the median nerve.

Step 5. Rehabilitation of the disabled patient. Wheelchairs and other aids and appliances can be used to reduce disability. Steps should be taken to preserve all aspects of the patient's life as much as possible. Successful management can make an enormous difference in the quality of lifeof rheumatoid patients.

Reference

1. Harrison's Principles of Internal Medicine – 13th Edition
2. Davidson's Principles of Practices of Medicine – 17th Edition

Question 269 Define infectious polyneuritis (Landry-Guillain-Barre syndrome).

Infectious polyneuritis (Landry-Guillain-Barre syndrome). It is a demyelinating neuropathy that usually follows 1-3 weeks after a viral infection, and the patients complain of the weakness ofthe distal limb muscles or distal numbness with an ascending weakness and areflexia and sensoryloss, and some patient with facial and respiratory muscles affected and the patient may be paralyzed.

Question 270 What is fibrositis syndrome?

Fibrositis syndrome. It is one of the most common rheumatic syndromes seen in women aged 20-50 with absent objective findings, and the investigations are normal. The patient may complain of musculoskeletal pain, fatigue, headaches, and numbness. Its cause is unknown, but sleep disorders, depression, and viral infection have been blamed. It may be a complication of hypothyroidism, rheumatoid arthritis, and sleep apnea. It may partially respond to exercise and amitriptyline.

Question 271 What complications may be associated with osteitis deformans (Paget's disease ofbone)?

Complications associated with osteitis deformans (Paget's disease of bone) 1. Deafness due tonerve compression. 2. High-output cardiac state from stunting. 3. Fracture through abnormal bone. 4. Paraplegia through vertebral involvement. 5. Osteogenic sarcoma.

Question 272-275 Differentiate between the childhood and facioscapulohumeral types of progressivemuscular dystrophy.

Progressive Muscular dystrophy

	Childhood	facioscapulohumeral
Inheritance	X-linked recessive	Autosomal dominant
Onset	4th year	10-40 years
Muscles affected	Proximal limbs weakness pseudohypertrophy of calveswith Gower's sign	Face, shoulder, pelvic girdle, pseudohypertrophy is rare
Progress	Severely disabled by 10 years old and death by 20 years old	Normal life expectancy slow progression

Question 276 What are the common causes of extracranial headaches?

Causes of extracranial headaches. 1. Tension headache. 2. Depression headache. 3. Cluster headache. 4. Temporal arteritis. 5. Cough headache. 6. Postherpetic neuralgia. 7. Others - dentalor ocular disease, temporomandibular joint dysfunction, sinusitis, hypertension, cervical spondylosis, and glaucoma.

Question 277 Define post-traumatic syndrome.

Post-traumatic syndrome. It is the vague complaints of headaches, dizziness, and malaise that follow minor to severe head injuries. Patients may have depression, and the symptoms may beprolonged.

Question 278 Outline the treatment of histamine headache.

Histamine headache. The patient can be given ergotamine tartrate aerosol, or inhalation of 100% oxygen (7 L/minute for 15 minutes) may be effective. Nasal spray butorphanol tartrate, a synthetic opioid agonist-antagonist, may also be effective.

Usually, oral drugs are not useful in this condition. Prophylactically, ergotaminetartrate can be given as rectal suppositories (0,5-1 mg at night or twice a day), by mouth (2 mgdaily), or by subcutaneous injection (0.25 mg three times daily for 5 days per week). Lithium carbonate and methysergide are also useful in the treatment. Propranolol and amitriptyline are found to be ineffective in treatment.

Question 279 Give the symptoms, management, and prevention of migraine headaches.

Migraine headache. Symptoms - The symptoms may be divided into

1 Migraine with aura. This last for 15 minutes to 1 hour or more. The patient experiences headaches, hemicrania, nausea, vomiting, and irritability. The superficial temporal arteryis engorged and pulsating. There may be patchy scotomata, unilateral blindness, hemianopia field loss, teichopsia, fortification spectra, and transient aphasia with tingling, numbness, or vague weakness of one side. The attack will cease after a few hours, followed by diuresis and sleep.

2. Migraine without aura. The patient may have a recurrent headache with nausea and malaise withvague visual symptoms.

3. Basilar migraine. Patients may present with circumoral tingling, tongue numbness,vertigo, diplopia, transient blindness, syncope, dysarthria, and ataxia.

4. Hemiplegic migraine. The patient will experience migraine with aura and hemiparesis. Recoveryoccurs within 24 hours.

5. Ophthalmoplegic migraine. The patient may have a third nerve palsy occurring in a migraineattack.

6. Facioplegic migraine. The patient may have a unilateral facial weakness during the migrainous attack.

Management During the acute attack. Patients may be tried first on simple analgesics with antiemetics, Sumatriptan, 5-hydroxytryptamine agonist by subcutaneous injection or orally can be given in recurrent severe attack Ergotamine tartrate (1-2 mg orally or rectally, 360 micrograms by aerosol or 0.25-0.5 mg by injection) may be useful if given early in the attack.

Prevention. Prophylactic drugs can be given to prevent a migrainous attack. Pizotifen, a 5- hydroxytryptamine antagonist, 0.5 mg at night for several days, increasing to 1,5 mg at night. Propranolol, 10 mg three times daily, increasing to 40-80 mg three times daily. Methysergide, a 5-hydroxytryptamine antagonist, 2-6 mg daily. Patients should stop oral contraceptives as they mayprecipitate a migrainous attack. Patients should be reassured and relieved of anxiety.

Question 280 What conditions predispose cerebral hemorrhage? What parts of the brain are mostliable to hemorrhage?

Conditions predisposing to cerebral hemorrhage.

1. Rupture of microaneurysm, especially in the patient with hypertension.
2. Saccular ("berry') aneurysms.
3. Arteriovenous malformations
4. Hemorrhage into cerebral infarct.
5. Hemorrhage into the cerebral tumor.
6. Rupture of the atheromatous vessel.
7. Rupture of mycotic aneurysm
8. Clotting disorders and anticoagulation.

Parts of the brain are most liable to hemorrhage. Basal ganglia, pons, cerebellum, and subcorticalwhite matter.

Question 281 Discuss the use of anticoagulants in

treating cerebral vascular accidents.

Use of anticoagulants in the treatment of cerebral vascular accidents (CVA). Indications for the use of anticoagulants in CVA are few and must be used discretely. 1. If there is a clear persistingembolic source, such as atrial fibrillation and dissection of the carotid artery. 2. Features of stroke in evolution over hours and days. 3. Certain cardiac valve lesions (uninfected) or cardiomyopathies. Urgent CT scan to rule out cerebral hemorrhage or tumor before starting anticoagulation. Anticoagulants are potentially dangerous in the 2 weeks following cerebral infarction because of the risk of provoking cerebral hemorrhage. Initial treatment should be withan intravenous infusion of heparin, and oral warfarin may be started at the same time, and the heparin has withdrawn after 3-4 days.

Question 282 Give the symptoms and signs of occlusion of the posterior inferior cerebellar artery.

Symptoms and signs of occlusion of the posterior inferior cerebellar artery. The patient would presentwith sudden vertigo and vomiting. There will be ipsilateral facial numbness, diplopia, nystagmus, ataxia, Horner's syndrome, and IY and Y nerve lesions. And the contralateral signs are the loss of pain, temperature sensation, and mild hemiparesis.

Question 283 What are the causes and symptoms of abscess of the brain?

Abscess of the brain.

Causes. Bacteria, e.g., streptococci, staphylococci, enterobacteria, fungi, and Bacteroides species may be introduced into the cerebral substances through:

1. Penetrating injury, e.g., fractures,

2. Direct spread through sinuses and middle ear,

3. Through embolism from systemic infection, such as bacterial endocarditis, pulmonary abscess

Symptoms. Patients may present with fever, headaches, meningism, and drowsiness which may occur over days and weeks.

Question 284 Give the clinical picture of cavernous sinus thrombosis.

Conditions predisposing to cerebral hemorrhage. 1. Rupture of microaneurysm, especially in the patient with hypertension. 2. Saccular ('berry') aneurysms. 3. Arteriovenous malformations 4. Hemorrhage into cerebral infarct. 5. Hemorrhage into the cerebral tumor. 6. Rupture of the atheromatous vessel. 7. Rupture of mycotic aneurysm 8. Clotting disorders and anticoagulation. Parts of the brain are most liable to hemorrhage. Basal ganglia, pons, cerebellum, and subcorticalwhite matter.

Question 285 What specific tests are commonly employed in the diagnosis of an intracranial tumors?

Tests in the diagnosis of intracranial tumors.

1. CT scan. CT scan only indicates the site of the mass, which could be benign or malignant tumors, cerebral abscesses, and cerebral infarction. The use of contrast enhancement may add to thediscriminating ability of CT when a mass is suspected.

2. MRI - is used to look especially for posterior fossa tumors.

3. Technetium brain scan - not a good discriminating test

but could be used to show lesion thatCT has missed.

4. Skull X-ray - may demonstrate changes in the dorsum sellae and clinoid process.
5. Others - angiography and ventriculography may be used to define a mass's site or blood supply.

Question 286 Differentiate the coma of opium poisoning from that of a cerebral hemorrhage.

Coma of opium poisoning. Patients may present with respiratory depression, convulsions, and pinpoint pupils. Investigation - drug screening.

Treatment with naloxone 0,8-2 mg intravenous is a competitive antagonist, and repeatedinjections may be required.

Coma of a cerebral hemorrhage. The patient may present with papilledema, epilepsy, dilatation of the pupil on the side of the lesion due to paresis of the sixth and third cranial nerves, and hemipareticsigns on the opposite side the lesion and incontinence.

Investigation - CT scan may show a cerebral hemorrhage. Treatment - treating the underlyingcause of the cerebral hemorrhage.

Question 287 Differentiate epilepsy from hysteria.

Epilepsy. It is a group of disorders with recurrent episodes of altered cerebral function associated with paroxysmal excessive and hypersynchronous discharge of cerebral neurons. The episodes of epilepsy vary from a brief lapse of awareness to prolonged bouts of unconsciousness, limb jerking, and incontinence. Causes - There is no clear cause in many cases. General epilepsy is secondary to a definable cause, e.g., anoxia or hypocalcemia. Partial epilepsy has a high incidence of the detectable cortical lesion. 40% of the cases may have a family historyof epilepsy. Clinical presentation Sleep deprivation, drugs, alcohol, and near TV screens may precipitate an attack of epilepsy. Patients may experience an aura moments before epilepsy with limb stiffening, jerking, automatisms, salivation, cyanosis, tongue biting, and incontinence and may have postictal symptoms like limb pain, headache, and drowsiness. Investigations.

Electroencephalography may help to establish and characterize the type of epilepsy; a CT scan isused to define or exclude a structural cause of epilepsy.

Treatment - to rule out if there are any organic causes of epilepsy and to treat its underlying cause. If there is an abnormal EEG, a strong family history, and no organic Causes can be found, the patient is treated with anticonvulsant drugs.

Hysteria It is where the patient's condition was results from unconscious psychological processes with poor insight into the nature of the symptoms and a maladaptive way of coping with a resolved psychological conflict. The role of organic causes is not well defined. Clinical presentation the patient may present with blindness, gait disturbance, loss of limb function, aphonia, pseudoseizures, and sensory loss. Dissociative amnesia is memory loss that is patchyand inconsistent with loss of identity and the tendency to travel aimlessly from home. Treatment - A full physical and psychiatric assessment is needed to identify the factors that may have precipitated the symptoms. Explanation of the symptoms and reassurance that the symptomswill get better is the initial treatment. In resistant cases, hypnosis or small doses of amylobarbitone may be helpful,

Question 288 Define catalepsy and give its etiology.

Catalepsy. It is a condition where the person's muscle tone is lost in the limbs, face, and trunk so that the person sinks to the ground and cannot move for seconds or minutes. There is no lossof consciousness, and EEG remains normal during the attack.

Etiology. Catalepsy is set off by surprise, emotion, laughter, fear, and embarrassment and whichmay have triggered the spontaneous activation of the REM sleep spinal inhibitory mechanism.

Question 289 Differentiate tonic and clonic spasms.

Tonic spasm. It is the rapid discharging of motor cortex cells causing tonic contractions ofmuscles with arms flexed and adducted and legs extended.

Clonic spasm It is the slower discharge of cortical cells with violent jerking of the face and limbswith tongue biting,

Question 290 What is the significance of the patellar reflex as a sign of disease?

Significance of patellar reflexes. Patellar reflexes are increased in upper motor neuron lesions.Patellar reflexes are decreased in lower motor neuron lesions. There is delayed relaxation of patellar reflexes in hypothyroidism.

Question 291 Outline the rehabilitation program of the hemiplegic.

The rehabilitation program of the hemiplegic. A skilled physiotherapist is essential in the first few months of the hemiplegic. It helps relieve spasticity, preventing contractures, and teaching stroke patients from using walking aids. A speech therapist is recommended for the hemiplegic with aphasia, the physiotherapy and speech therapy have psychological importance for the hemiplegic. A visit to the patient's home by the occupational therapist and the primary physician to discuss modifications to the pattern of the lifestyle of the hemiplegic at home, such as stair rails, portable lavatories, bath rails, hoists, sliding boards, wheelchairs, tripods, modificationof doorways and sleep arrangements, stair lifts, and kitchen modifications.

Question 292 Discuss the treatment of epilepsy.

Treatment of epilepsy.

A. Emergency treatment. To ensure that the patients harm themselves as little as possible and that the airway is patent in a prolonged seizure and in a postictal coma. A prolonged or repeated seizure outside the hospital is best treated with diazepam solution (10 mg). Status epilepticus is when seizures follow each other without recovery, and there is a serious risk of deathdue to respiratory failure. Treatment with immediate intravenous injection of diazepam 10 mg followed by intravenous infusion of 200 mg/liter over 24 hours and with ventilatory support. If status epilepticus continues or returns, chlormethiazole 0.8% should be given by intravenous infusion.

B. Anticonvulsant drug treatment. It is used for recurrent seizures. The commonly used drugs arephenytoin 300 mg in divided doses, carbamazepine 200 mg three times daily, and sodium valproate 200 mg times daily. Phenytoin could be used for generalized tonic-clonic seizures, sodium valproate for generalized absence and partial seizures, and carbamazepine for partial seizures. Using one drug alone in the treatment is preferable, and a second drug may be used in resistant cases. Vigabatrin and lamotrigine may be used in resistant cases.

C. Neurosurgical treatment. Amputation of the anterior temporal lobe, usually for the non-dominant side in patients with partial seizures or partial seizures, may be one of the several surgical treatments for seizures.

D. Pregnancy and epilepsy. Regular monitoring of drug levels is required as fits are more common in pregnancy due to poor absorption and poor compliance with drug therapy. Breastfeeding is only contraindicated with patients on phenobarbitone or primidone.

E Social implication of epilepsy. Adults and children with epilepsy are encouraged to lead unrestricted lives. Advise for these patients, such as avoiding swimming alone and dangerous sports like rock climbing or solo canoeing, and confer to the driving regulations in that area.

Question 293 Describe aphasia.

Aphasia. It is the loss or defect in language caused by left front temporoparietal lesions.

Broca's aphasia. The expressive aphasia due to a lesion in the left frontal lobe caused reduced fluency of speech with comprehension relatively preserved.

2. Wernicke's aphasia. The receptive aphasia is due to a left temporoparietal lesion leaving afluent language, but the words themselves are incorrect.

3. Nominal aphasia. There is difficulty in naming familiar objects and is due to a left posterior temporal/inferior parietal lesion,

4. Global aphasia. It is an expressive disturbance characteristic of Broca's aphasia and the loss of comprehension of Wernicke's aphasia, and it is due to a severe left hemisphere infarct with writing and reading affected.

Question 294 Outline the treatment of parkinsonism (postencephalitic, idiopathic and arteriosclerotic).

Treatment of Parkinsonism.

Drug treatment. Levodopa in combination with a peripheral decarboxylase inhibitor, benserazide(co-beneldopa), or carbidopa (co-careldopa). This combination treatment reduces the peripheral side effects like nausea and increases the availability of the dopamine component in the central nervous system. Treatment is started gradually with co-beneldopa 125 mg or co-careldopa one tablet three times daily and increased until either an adequate improvement has taken place or side-effects limit further increase in dose. Fluctuation in response to levodopa may occur. The duration of the action of the drug may contract, and the patient begins to suffer from chronic levodopa syndrome. That is patient's condition fluctuates between dopa-induced dyskinesias (chorea and dystonic movements) and severe and sometimes sudden immobility (on-off syndrome). Periods of drug withdrawal may be helpful and close supervision of patients as therecould be severe rigidity and akinesia following the withdrawal of levodopa.

Physiotherapy and physical aids. A skilled physiotherapist

can improve the gait and help the patient to overcome problems such as a. Clothing - avoid zips, fiddly buttons, and lace-up shoes. b. Cutlery - use built-up handles. c. Chairs - high, upright chairs are easier to rise from than deep comfortable armchairs. d. Rails - should be fixed near the lavatory and baths. e. Shoes - should be easy to put on and have smooth soles. f. Flooring - Patient may prefer to walk onvinyl or linoleum, g. Walking aids - a frame or a tripod.

Question 295 Define and list the common causes of syncope.

Syncope. It is the loss of consciousness resulting from an inadequate blood supply to the braindue to sudden reflex bradycardia and peripheral and splanchnic vasodilatation

Causes.

1 Vasovagal or neurocardiogenic syncope. Due to prolonged standing, fear, pain, micturition orcoughing.
2 Simple syncope. Common in childhood, youth, or pregnancy.
3. Syndrome of carotid sinus syncope. Common in the elderly and is due to increased carotid sinussensitivity to external pressure.
4. Postural hypotension. Due to vasodilator and antihypertensive drugs.
5. Cardiac syncope due to: Diminished cardiac output from complete heart block. Very rapidtachycardias - ventricular tachycardias and ventricular fibrillation. Exertional syncope from severe left ventricular outflow obstruction (aortic stenosis).
6. Transient cerebral ischemia due to cervical spondylosis where vertebral artery compressionoccurs.

Question 296 Give a short outline of the symptomatology of dementia paralytica.

Symptomatology of dementia paralytica. The patient may present with disturbance of memory, thinking, orientation, comprehension, language, and judgment with no clouding of consciousness but with the presence of weakness, tremors, brisk reflexes, and extensor plantar reflexes. There maybe a progressive dementia, and seizures may occur.

Question 297 Give the symptoms and treatment of tabes dorsalis.

Symptoms of tabes dorsalis. Paresthesia or recurrent shooting pain in the muscles of the leg. Impairment of proprioception and vibration sense. Argyll Robertson pupils. Sharp abdominalpain with nausea and vomiting. Paroxysmal cough and dyspnea. Painful bladder spasms.
Neuropathic joints (Charcot's joints) Treatment. Aqueous crystalline penicillin G, 2-4 millionunits intravenously every 4 hours for 10-14 days, or 2-4 million units of procaine penicillin intramuscularly once a day along with 500 mg of probenecid orally four times daily for 10-14days.

Question 298 What are the causes, symptoms, and prognosis of Bell's palsy?

Bell's palsy.

Causes. It is caused by a viral infection that causes swelling of the nerve within the petroustemporal bone resulting in an acute isolated facial nerve palsy.

Symptoms. The patient may have a marked unilateral facial weakness with loss of taste on the anterior two-thirds of the tongue. There may be some pain behind the ear.

Prognosis. Many patients have marked improvement towards the end of the second week, but recovery may take up to 12 months to be complete. About 15% of the patients are left with severe, unsightly residual weakness.

Question 299 Give the treatment of trigeminal neuralgia (tic douloureux).

Treatment of trigeminal neuralgia (tic douloureux). Carbamazepine 600-1200 mg daily may suppress the pain in the majority of cases. Alcohol injection into the trigeminal ganglion or peripheral fifth nerve branches. Surgical procedures may be carried out if drug therapy fails, suchas radiofrequency extirpation of the ganglion, nerve decompression, or sectioning of the sensory root.

Question 300 What is Horner's syndrome?

Homer's syndrome. It is due to a lesion of the sympathetic pathway on the same side. Patients present with unilateral pupillary constriction with slight relative ptosis and enophthalmos. Thereis a loss of sweating on the same side of the face or body.

Causes of Horner's syndrome. 1 Hemisphere and brain stem lesions. Massive cerebral infarction,pontine glioma, lateral medullary syndrome, and 'coming' of the temporal lobe 2. Cervical cord lesions. Syringomyelia and cord tumors. 3. Tl root lesions. Bronchial neoplasm (apical), apical tuberculosis, cervical rib, and brachial plexus trauma, 4. Sympathetic chain in the neck. Following thyroid/laryngeal surgery, carotid artery occlusion, neoplastic infiltration, cervical sympathectomy.

Question 301 Give the common causes of vertigo.

Causes of vertigo. 1. Meniere's disease. 2. Drugs - e.g. gentamicin, anticonvulsant intoxication.
3. Toxins - e.g., ethyl alcohol 4. Vestibular neuronitis S. Multiple sclerosis. 6. Migraine. 7. Acutecerebellar lesions. 8. Cerebellopontine angle lesions. 9. Partial seizures 10. Brain stem ischemia or infarction. 11. Benign positional vertigo.

Question 302 What is the most common cause of a choked disk?

The most common cause of choked disks is idiopathic intracranial hypertension or benign intracranial hypertension.

Question 303 Differentiate between Meniere's syndrome and brain tumor.

Meniere's syndrome. It is due to dilatation of ht c endolymph system and is characterized by recurrent attacks of vertigo, tinnitus, and deafness. The patient presents with sudden attacks of vertigo with vomiting and loss of balance, and the attacks are recurrent over months and years.Nystagmus and sensorineural deafness may be present.

Brain tumor Brain tumors account for 2% of deaths; the majority are benign and malignant tumors arising within the central nervous system, and the remainder is metastatic tumors. The patients present with signs of raised intracranial pressure: headache, impairment of consciousness, papilledema, vomiting, and bradycardia.

There may be epilepsy and local effects on adjacent cerebral tissue due to the brain tumor.

Question 304 Describe the gait associated with cerebellar disease.

<u>Gait associated with cerebellar disease.</u>

Disease of the lateral lobes of the cerebellum. The patient's stance is broad-based, unstable, and tremulous. The gait tends to veer towards the side of the more affected cerebellar lobe.

B. Diseases of the cerebellar vermis. The patient's trunk becomes unsteady, and there is a tendency tofall backward.

Question 305 What is the significance of the absence of abdominal reflexes?

Significance of the absence of abdominal reflexes. The abdominal reflexes are cutaneous reflexes mediated through a spinal reflex arc, and its abdominal responses are notoriously variable. The abdominal can be diminished or absent in old age, obese patients, and women who have had children.

Question 306 Discuss the diagnosis of amyotrophic lateral sclerosis.

<u>Diagnosis of amyotrophic lateral sclerosis</u>. There are no specific diagnostic tests, and the diagnosis is usually made on clinical grounds. Wasting of the muscles begins in the small muscles of one hand, spreads throughout the arm, and soon follows on the other side. Wasting and weakness with fasciculation of the muscles and the tendon reflexes are exaggerated. As the disease progresses, there would be

spastic tetraparesis or paraparesis with added lower motor neuron signs. There would be a mixture of upper motor neuron and lower motor neuron signs, e.g., awasted fibrillating tongue with a spastic weak palate. The patient may have dysarthria, dysphagia, nasal fluids regurgitation, and choking. The patient's awareness, ocular movements, and cerebellar or extrapyramidal signs are preserved. Electromyography may show chronic partial denervation with preserved motor conduction velocity. The cerebrospinal fluid examination is usually normal, and sometimes the protein may be slightly raised.

Question 307. Describe the symptoms and treatment of hydrocephalus in children.

Hydrocephalus in children.

Symptoms. The patient may present with nonspecific symptoms like headaches that are variable in location and intensity occasionally occurring early in the morning associated with vomiting. Personality and behavior changes, including irritability or indifference, are sometimes noted.
Lethargy and drowsiness are relatively late symptoms. Nausea and vomiting are secondary to increased intracranial pressure, particularly in the posterior fossa.

Treatment. 1. Specific treatment for any underlying hydrocephalus-related conditions, such as brain tumors, abscesses, and chronic meningitis. 2. Surgery is the most effective means of treating progressive hydrocephalus, and a shunt between the cerebral ventricles and the peritoneal cavity is the most employed surgical technique. This shunt allows for diverting cerebrospinal fluid into the peritoneal cavity, where it is absorbed as a palliative measure and not a cure. 3. Medical treatment using agents like acetazolamide, furosemide, and glycerol can decrease cerebrospinal fluid production, and it is used when the hydrocephalus is slowly progressive and perhaps transitory. It may also be used during the interim period when an infectedshunt system has to be removed and before a new system can be inserted.

Question 309 Discuss symptomatology and diagnosis of multiple sclerosis.

Symptoms. The patient complains of blurring of vision in one eye and mild ocular pain, and thesymptoms may progress over days to produce severe visual loss. Recovery may occur within amonth. Involvement of the brain stem may produce diplopia, vertigo, facial numbness or dysphagia but without tinnitus or deafness, which may last for weeks before recovery.
Demyelination of the cord will cause spastic paraparesis, difficulty walking, sensory disturbance, and urinary symptoms. Tonic spasms or brief spasms of the limb or even epilepsy is common. In the end stage of the disease, there may be a combination of spastic tetraparesis, ataxia, optic atrophy, nystagmus, brain stem signs, pseudobulbar palsy, incontinence of urine, and dementia.

Diagnosis.

1. MRI of the brain is the gold-standard investigation - multiple plaques are visible in the periventricular region and brain stem.
2. There may be the presence of oligoclonal bands of IgG in the cerebrospinal fluid examination.
3. There may be a delay in the visual-evoked response (VER).

Question 310 Give the symptoms and management of acute chorea (St. Vitus' dance, Sydenham'schorea).

Symptoms of acute chorea. It occurs in cases of rheumatic fever, during pregnancy, orin those taking oral contraceptives. The onset of the chorea is gradual and sometimes with confusion. There would be irritability, insolence and inattentiveness herald the onset of fidgety movements, which is sometimes predominantly unilateral.

Management. Sedation and dopamine receptor antagonists, such as phenothiazines or butyrophenones, such as haloperidol 0.5-1.5 mg 8-hourly or dopamine-depleting agents, such astetrabenazine 25-50 mg 8-hourly may be used to control the acute chorea.

Treatment of the underlying cause of acute chorea with phenoxymethylpenicillin 250-500 mg 8-hourly for at least 5 years.

Question 311 Discuss the classifications of mental disorders.

Classification of mental disorders. A. Organic psychiatric disorders. 1. Acute - e.g., delirium 2.Chronic - e.g., dementia B. Schizophrenia C. Affective disorders 1. Depression 2. Mania 3.
Recurrent affective disorders D. Neurotic, stress-related and somatoform disorders 1. Anxiety disorders - generalized anxiety, phobic anxiety, panic disorder 2. Obsessive-compulsive disorder 3. Reaction to severe stress - acute stress disorder, post-traumatic stress disorder, adjustmentdisorder. 4. Dissociative disorder 5. Somatoform disorder 6. Neurasthenia E. Behavioral syndromes 1. Eating disorders 2. Sleep disorders 3. Sexual

dysfunction 4. Puerperal mental disorder E. Personality disorders G. Substance misuse - alcohol abuse, drug abuse H. Psychosexual disorders - sexual dysfunction, sexual deviations, gender role disorders.

Question 312 Discuss the terms psychosis and psychoneurosis.

Psychosis. It is a term used to imply a psychiatric disorder that significantly impairs insight, involves a substantial break with reality, has a major impact on the individual's personalityand functioning, and may require specialized inpatient treatment. Some of the psychotic symptoms like delusions, hallucinations, and formal disorder.

Psychoneurosis. It is a term used in psychiatric disorders in which psychotic symptoms and features are absent, the patient's personality is relatively undamaged, and contact with reality is unimpaired. It can be thought of as an exaggerated form of normal reactions to stressful events, such as anxiety, depression, irritability, and physical symptoms lacking an organic cause.

Question 313 Mention some characteristics of mental or emotional pain (psychalgia) which wouldaid in its differentiation from bodily pain or solastalgia.

Characteristics of mental or emotional pain (psychalgia).

1. The patient presents with severe, persistent pain, which a physical illness or psychological disturbance cannot explain.
2. There would be sufficient emotional conflicts or psychosocial problems which influence thepain.
3. Patients would usually demand emotional support from their families and treatment from their medical doctors.

Question 314 Give four examples of psychoneurosis.

Examples of psychoneurosis. 1. Anxiety neurosis. 2. Hysterical neurosis. 3. Hypochondriacalneurosis. 4. Obsessional neurosis

Question 315 Define and differentiate illusion, delusion, and hallucination.

Illusion. It is the misperception of external stimuli and is most likely to occur when the generallevel of sensory stimulation is reduced.

Delusion. It is defined as an abnormal belief arising from distorted judgments that is held with absolute conviction, not amenable to reason or modifiable by experience, and experienced asa self-evident truth of great personal significance.

Hallucination It is defined as a thorough conviction of a sensation when no external object to excite or provoke such a sensation is present, and that is perceived as having qualities of normal perceptions and independent of the individual's will.

Question 316 What are the character traits of individuals classified as pathologic without actualmental disorders? Give some examples.

Character traits of individuals classified as pathologic without actual mental disorders. Patientswith pathological diseases with psychiatric symptoms are:

A. Depression - carcinoma, thyroid disorders, diabetes mellitus.

B. Anxiety - hyperthyroidism, hypoglycemia, alcohol/drug withdrawal

C. Irritability - head injury, hypoglycemia, premenstrual tension

D. Fatigue - anemia, sleep disorders, carcinoma.

References

1. Harrison's Principles of Internal Medicine – 13th Edition
2. Davidson's Principles of Practices of Medicine – 17th Edition

Question 317 What is combat fatigue?

Combat fatigue. The patient would present with fatigue, poor concentration and memory, irritability, alteration in sleep, and muscular aches. It may be due to a viral infection, and the investigations are usually normal.

Question 318 Outline the causes and treatment of insomnia.

Causes of insomnia.

1. Common causes - Stress, caffeine, physical discomfort, daytime napping, and early bedtime.
2. Depression.
3. Manic disorders,
4. Abuse of alcohol.
5. Heavy smoking.
6. Medical conditions - pain, delirium, respiratory distress syndrome, uremia, asthma, and hypothyroidism.

Treatment.

1. Educating the patients about regular exercise, healthy

sleep, avoiding heavy meals, alcoholand caffeine-containing drinks in the evening

2. Treat the underlying causes, and if necessary, anti-depressive or antipsychotic drugs withsedative effects, e.g., trazodone or thioridazine, may be used for a short course.
3. For acute distress, patients may use a short course of benzodiazepine, e.g., temazepam 15 mgat bedtime, or antihistamine, e.g., diphenhydramine.

Question 319 Outline the management of psychoneurosis.

Management of psychoneurosis.

A. Medical measures. All underlying medical disorders which cause psychoneurosis must be ruled out and treated. Patients with generalized anxiety may be treated with benzodiazepines and buspirone, which are anxiolytics of choice. Patients with panic attacks may be treated with a paper bag used for rebreathing in hyperventilation episodes. Antidepressants are the initial drug ofchoice. Clonazepam and alprazolam are alternatives to antidepressants. Fluoxetine is effective in attacks associated with obsessive-compulsive disorder. The phobic disorder may be treated with MAO inhibitors or fluoxetine. Moderate doses of beta-blockers may be used for phobias likeperformance anxiety. Patients with obsessive-compulsive disorders may be treated with clomipramine and fluoxetine.

B. Behavioral measures. Relaxation techniques can sometimes help reduce anxiety.Exposing the patient to graded doses of a phobic object or situation is desensitization.

C. Psychologic measures. Cognitive approaches are

effective in the treatment of panic disorders, phobias, and obsessive-compulsive disorders. A combination of medical and cognitive therapy is more effective than either alone. Group therapy is the treatment of choice when anxiety isthe patient's difficulties in dealing with others.

D. Social measures. Family counseling to aid acceptance of the patient's symptoms. Maintainingthe social structure is anxiety-alleviating, and work, school and social activities should be maintained.

Question 320 What is understood by the term " epilepsies"? Give the treatment of epileptic psychosis.

The epilepsies. It is a term used to classify localization-related and generalized epilepsies. A. Localization-related epilepsies.

1. Idiopathic, with age-related onset. a. Benign childhood epilepsy with the centrotemporal spike. b.Childhood epilepsy with occipital paroxysms.
2. Symptomatic - syndromes of great individual variability based on anatomic locale clinicalfeatures, seizure types, and etiologic factors.

B. Generalized epilepsies.

1. Idiopathic, with age-related onset. a. Benign neonatal familial convulsions. b. Benign neonatalconvulsions. c. Benign myoclonic epilepsy in infancy d. Childhood absence epilepsy (pyknolepsy) e. Juvenile absence epilepsy. f. Juvenile myoclonic epilepsy (impulsive petit mal)

g. Epilepsy with grand mal seizures (GTCS) on awakening.

2. Idiopathic and/or symptomatic a. West syndrome (infantile spasms) b. Lennox-Gas taut syndrome c. Epilepsy with myoclonic-astatic seizures d. Epilepsy with myoclonic absences 3. Symptomatic a. Nonspecific etiology - early myoclonic encephalopathy. b. Specific syndromes-epileptic seizures may complicate many diseases.

Treatment of epileptic psychosis.

Patients may be treated with carbamazepine 200 mg three times daily or phenytoin 300 mg daily or sodium valproate 200 mg three times daily with monitoring of the plasma drug levels.

Reference

1. Harrison's Principles of Internal Medicine – 13th Edition
2. Davidson's Principles of Practices of Medicine – 17th Edition

Question 321 Mention and define a psychosis with a definite alcoholic etiology.

Psychosis with a definite alcoholic etiology.

Alcohol dependence syndrome is a psychiatric disorder which consists of:

1. The compulsive need to drink.
2. Drink at regular intervals to avoid and relieve withdrawal symptoms.
3. Increasing tolerance is an important sign of increasing dependence.
4. Repeated withdrawal symptoms.
5. The patient will take a drink in the morning to stave off

withdrawal symptoms.

6. Reinstatement of drinking after a period of abstinence.

Question 322 What is involutional melancholia?

Involutional melancholia. It is a postmenopausal depression, where a patient may have severeagitation and psychotic ideation ranging from general suspicion to ideas of references with delusions.

Question 323 Give a brief description of paranoia.

Paranoia These patients are very sensitive to criticism and humiliation. They are excessively keen on establishing what they regard as their personal rights and defending them forcefully. Theycan be very suspicious and would blame others for their own mistakes. This is apparent when they get medically sick and would blame the doctor for negligence or bad practice.

Question 324 Discuss the psychotic features of general paresis and methods of treatment.

Psychotic features of general paresis.

Patients may have a delusion of grandeur, confusion, irresponsible, slovenly, and psychotic. There maybe also a decrease in concentration, memory loss, irritability, and mild headache.

Treatment. Injection of procaine penicillin 600-1200 mg daily for 3 weeks. Further courses ofpenicillin must be given if symptoms are not relieved or the conditions continue to advance

Question 325 Describe and give the treatment of

schizophrenia.

There is no definite cause of schizophrenia. However, some of the possible biological causes are:

Genetic. 40% risk for children of two affected parents. 50% risk for the monozygotic twin of the affected individual.

1. Dopamine agonists, e.g., amphetamine, exacerbate the condition, and withdrawal of dopamineantagonists cause a rebound of symptoms in some patients.

2. Brain damage, e.g., in utero from a long-acting virus, may result in the enlargement of lateral ventricles and widening of cerebral fissures and sulci on CT scans.

Clinical features

The peak age of onset is in late adolescence and in the early twenties. The overall sex incidence is about equal. The symptoms consist of 1. Auditory hallucinations - patients hear their thoughts spoken aloud and can hear one or several voices referring to themselves in the third person or referring to them by name, or hearing voices commenting on their behavior. 2. Thoughts withdrawal, insertion, and interruption. 3. Thought broadcasting. 4. Delusional perceptions. 5. External control of emotions. 6. Somatic passivity and feelings - patients believe that thoughts oracts are due to the influence of others. Chronic schizophrenia is characterized by thought disorder, lack of drive, social withdrawal, emotional emptiness, catatonia, and delusions.

Good prognostic factors.

1. No family history of schizophrenia.
2. Stable personality and stable home relationship.

3. Identifiable precipitating factor and acute onset.
4. Prompt treatment.

Poor prognostic factors.

1. Family history of schizophrenia.
2. Withdrawal, solitary, eccentric personality, and stormy domestic situation.
3. Insidious onset and no identifiable triggering factors.
4. Delayed treatment.

Treatment.

Medical measures. Phenothiazines are used, and it may take up to 3 months for complete controlof positive symptoms, and premature discontinuation of treatment may result in prompt relapse.

Chlorpromazine 100-1000 mg daily in the drug of choice if sedation is required. Trifluoperazine is used if sedation is undesirable. Fluphenazine deaconate 25-100 mg intramuscular every 1-4 weeks for long-term prophylactic toprevent relapse Clozapine is used in patients with intractable schizophrenia.

Social measures.

Treatment of psychiatric patients should be a multi-disciplinary approach involving psychiatrists, psychiatric nurses, psychologists, psychiatric social workers, Psychiatric community nurses, occupational therapists, and counselors. Patients would require rehabilitationin a structured work and social environment. Parents and relatives need advice concerning the optimum amount of emotional and social stimulation to be provided for the patient. Severely disabled patients require long-term residential medical and nursing care.

Question 326 Give a brief general description of maniac-depressive psychosis, including etiology and treatment.

Maniac-depressive psychosis.

The possible etiological factors are:

1. Genetic. 10-15% of first-degree relatives have an affective disorder. 68% of monozygotictwins reared together or apart are concordant for manic depressive disorder.
2. Biochemical Imbalance of neurotransmitters, e.g., monoamine neurotransmitters, are depletedin depression but increased in mania. Hormonal factors, e.g., depression, is more common afterchildbirth, in the premenstrual phase, with the use of oral contraceptives, menopause, and post hysterectomy.
3. Maternal deprivation - loss of early maternal affection in early life predisposes a person toaffective disorder in later life.
4. Stressful events - bereavement, loss of a job, moving to a new house, and marriage.

Clinical features the patients may be in the normal mood or a marked elevated mood (mania) or indepression.

Features of mania:

1. Mood - elevated, infectious, labile
2. Talk - fast, pressurized, flight of ideas
3. Energy - excessive, restless, distractible
4. Ideation - grandiose, self-confident, delusions of wealth, power, influence, or of religioussignificance,

persecutory delusions.

5. The cognition-formal testing difficulty, disturbance of retrieval of memories.

6. Physical - insomnia, mild to moderate weight loss 7. Behavior - disinhibition, increased sexualinterest, excessive drinking or spending 8. Hallucinations - fleeting auditory or visual

Features of depression.

1. Mood - depressed, miserable, unhappy
2. Talk - impoverished, slow monotonous, incomplete
3. Energy - lacking, retarded, apathetic
4. Ideation - feelings of futility, guilt, self-reproach, unworthiness, hypochondriacal preoccupations, worrying, suicidal thoughts, the delusion of guilt, nihilism, and persecution.
5. Cognition – verbal memory impaired, pseudodementia is elderly.
6. Physical - early waking, appetite, and weight loss, constipation, loss of libido, impotence, fatigue, bodily aches, and pains.
7. Behavior - retardation or agitation, poverty of movement andexpression. 8. Hallucinations - auditory, which is hostile and critical.

Treatment

Simple support, reassurance, sympathy, and the opportunity to express distress and negative feelings are often enough to bring about relief from a minor depressive illness. However, hospitalization isusually necessary in cases of severe depression, suicidal patients, and mania.

A. Treatment of depression.

1. Tricyclic antidepressants. Imipramine and amitriptyline,

orally 25-75 mg daily and increasingto 150-200 mg over a week. It takes 2-3 weeks for the full therapeutic effect. Other tricyclics used are nortriptyline, doxepin, and mianserin.

2. Serotonin uptake inhibitors. Fluoxetine and paroxetine produce less side effects and the speedie ronset of therapeutic effects.

3. Monoamine oxidase inhibitors - are used in depressions where the patients present with marked anxiety and obsessional or hypochondriacal features. Phenelzine 30-60 mg daily is widely used.Moclobemide 300 mg daily, newer forms of MAOI.

4. Electroconvulsive therapy. It is a treatment of choice where:

- The patient is dangerously suicidal
- A delay in treatment represents a serious risk to health.
- The patient is refusing food and drink.
- The patient is in a depressive stupor.

A course of 6-8 treatments over 3 weeks may be used in severe depression characterized byretardation and delusions.

B. Treatment of mania

Acute attacks are treated with chlorpromazine, haloperidol, and pimozide, and treatment may be required for up to 3 months. Prophylactic treatment with lithium carbonate for the patient with repeated mania and/or depression attacks. Lithium takes at least 10 days to take effect, and thelithium levels and the thyroid and renal functions should be checked every 3-4 months. Carbamazepine used in prophylaxis for maniac cases. A combination of lithium and carbamazepine may be more effective than either drug alone.

C. Psychological treatment.

Supportive – sympathy, reassurance, and information should be part of every patient's treatment. Cognitive therapy – this behavioral therapy combines behavioral tasks with questioning and arguments designed to alter some of the ideas that are common among depressed patients and that appear to prolong their depression.

References I

1. Harrison's Principles of Internal Medicine – 13th Edition
2. Davidson's Principles of Practices of Medicine – 17th Edition

Appendix 1

Appendix II: Comments

Appendix II (b):

Appendix III: Ancillary Comments

Appendix IV: Comments on Various

Benjamin Alli, MD, Ph.D., is a Sakellarides Professor of Medicine and Surgery and the Chancellor of the Royal College of Physicians and Surgeons of the United States of America.

References II:

1. American Academy of Neurology. (2019, April 30). *Cannabis-based medicine may reduce seizures for children with difficult-to-Treat epilepsy*. PR Newswire: press releasedistribution, targeting, monitoring and marketing. https://www.prnewswire.com/news-releases/cannabis-based-medicine-may-reduce-seizures-for-children-with-difficult-to-treat-epilepsy-300841365.html

2. Billiamin A. Alli, (n.d.). National Center for Biotechnology Information. https://www.ncbi.nlm.nih.gov/pmc/articles/PMC2536916/pdf/jnma00009-0039.pdf

3. Billiamin A. Alli, (n.d.). National Center for Biotechnology Information. https://www.ncbi.nlm.nih.gov/pmc/articles/PMC2537146/pdf/jnma00017-0059.pdf

Made in the USA
Monee, IL
13 May 2025

17411780R00144